Healing Secrets

Of

Ancient China

Pier Tsui-Po

First published in Australia 1994
by Hill of Content Publishing Co Pty Ltd
86 Bourke Street Melbourne 3000 Australia

Cover design: Todd Davidson
Format and Design: Hicks Alexander & Associates
Printed by: Australian Print Group, Maryborough, Victoria

National Library of Australia
Cataloguing-in-Publication data

Tsui-Po, Pier, 1954-
  Healing secrets of ancient China

Bibliography.
ISBN 0 85572 245 2.

1. Medicine, Chinese. 2. Taoism. 3. Medicine, Chinese-Philosophy. 4. Mind
and Body. I. Title

610.951

The author and publisher wishes to express their thanks and appreciation to the
following who granted permission to quote from:

The Elements of Taoism by Martin Palmer.
Publisher: Element Books Limited, Shaftesbury, Dorset, England.

Yellow Emperor's Classic of Internal Medicine by Ilza Veith.
Publisher: University of California Press, California, USA.

Dedicated to my late father, Xiong,

my mother, Elda

and my wife, Sally,

for their love and support.

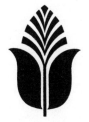

*'Yet it is said: Those who have the true wisdom remain strong
while those who have no knowledge and wisdom grow old and
feeble. Therefore the people should share this wisdom and their
names will become famous. Those who are wise inquire and
search together, while those who are ignorant and stupid
inquire and search apart from each other. Those who are stupid
and ignorant do not exert themselves enough in the search for
the Right Way, while those who are wise search beyond the
natural limits.*

*Those who search beyond the natural limits will retain good
hearing and clear vision, their bodies will remain light and
strong, and although they grow old in years they will remain
able-bodied and flourishing; and those who are able-bodied
can govern to great advantage.'*

The Yellow Emperor's Classic of Internal Medicine, the oldest,
most widely used Chinese medical classic is the source of
traditional Chinese medical science. It was first published circa
100 BC in ancient China.

(Translation by Ilza Veith, 1972, p. 121.)

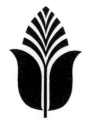

Contents

Acknowledgements

My special thanks to: all my teachers without whom this work would not have been possible; Charles Tsui-Po, Richard Tsui-Po and Steeve Kiat for maintaining Golden Lion's high standards; Allan Hall for his assistance and thorough understanding of my philosophy; Allan Hicks for his computer expertise in designing and formatting the layout of the book; Trevor Phillips for photography; Margaret Hicks, my mother-in-law, for rescuing me from my household chores; Bin Cong for his help with Chinese translations; and to all students of the Golden Lion Academy for their encouragement.

Author's note

Man

This expression is used throughout the book to denote human beings, both of male and female gender. The author does not imply discrimination of any kind at all in the use of this term.

Capitals

Some terms such as Chi, Yin and Yang are specific concepts in Chinese culture and they have no accurate English equivalent. Therefore, I have chosen to refer to them in transliterated Chinese throughout the book.

Including these words, there are also other words and concepts such as Wind or Liver Yang that indicate a specific Chinese medical disease state. They have little or no resemblance to their meanings in the English language. Therefore I have capitalised some English words to account for their special meaning.

Transliteration

Conventional spellings based on the Wade-Giles system for some familiar terms and names such as Chi and Huang Ti have been retained in order to correlate to the transliteration of the texts used as reference.

It should be pointed out that the Pinyin method of transliteration is now used throughout the world. In this book both systems are used. Therefore I have included the following table for terms that are not in Pinyin romanisation. The closest English sounds of some key words are also extended to help you pronounce them.

Wade-Giles	Pinyin	Closest English Sound
Lao	Lao	as in Loud
Tsu	Tzu	as in Zoo
Tao	Dao	as in Dowry
Te	De	as in Dermot
Ching	Jing	as in Jingle
Yin	Yin	as in Yin
Yang	Yang	as in Yeang
Chi	Qi	as in Cheese
Huang	Huang	as in Whung
Ti	Di	as in Dee
Nei	Nei	as in Neighbour
Tai Chi	Tai Ji	as in Tie Chee
Kung Fu	Gong Fu	as in Goong Foo
Chi Kung	Qi Qong	as in Chee Goong

Introduction

Let us explore the beginning...
...when time appeared to stand still
...when the land was pure
...when man lived in harmony with nature.

Behind and within everything in the Universe is a force and potential called Tao or 'the way'. The ideal life for each individual person, order for society and harmony in nature is based upon and guided by the Tao.

The ancient art of Taoism is the essence upon which the healing secrets of ancient China are founded. It also forms the basis of the Chinese philosophy of life.

Tao is the ultimate source of all, the beginning before the beginning and the uncreated which constantly creates everything. Tao has influence over all things and creation is a result of Tao.

In ancient times, mankind thrived by living naturally. The purity of life in those early days produced great philosophers, sages, and spiritual leaders such as Lao Tsu, Yellow Emperor, Buddha, and Confucius. Their teachings were based on the natural laws of the Universe.

Their original works taught that Man, in his absolute dependence, could do no better than to follow a way conceived after that of Nature. They saw the Universe endowed with a spirit that is generous to those who follow it and unforgiving to those who do not.

They also perceived that within nature there was a graduation of power. The Earth was dependent on Heaven, and man was dependent on both Heaven and Earth. When rain did not come or when the winter snow thawed too late for young animals, Heaven was more powerful. Heaven, through its material manifestations, was the ruler of the world. It unites its Tao with that of the Earth in order to complete the yearly cycle of nature. This synergy between fundamental powers allowed mankind to easily conform with and benefit from the way of Tao.

Lao Tsu, meaning old philosopher, was a native of Chu (in modern Henan province). His given name was Li Erh and he was a custodian of the Imperial Archives. When he retired, he was asked by the gate keeper of the Imperial Palace to write his philosophy of life gained through his years of studying the Imperial records and manuscripts. Hence Tao Te Ching (formerly called Lao Tsu's book) was born. Its impact on Chinese civilisation, culture and healing is beyond description.

There are more commentaries and English translations of the Tao Te Ching than any other book, except the Bible. Due to the vagaries of the Chinese language when compared to English, it is possible to translate any given Chinese text into a large number of interpretations. I have chosen to rely on my own personal translation of Lao Tsu's *Tao Te Ching* as taught to me by my instructors.

Lao Tsu believed that some artifacts of man led to evil and destruction. He taught that man must follow the Tao to find peace and contentment. For when Man is completely in tune with himself and the Universe that surrounds him, when his actions and the actions of the Universe are one, then Man will have realised his infinite nature.

The beginning of Taoism marked a philosophical turning point in the changing condition of the times when poverty, starvation, ignorance, greed, exploitation, war, killings and unprincipled rulers affected humans and the Universe in much the same way they do today.

...Man stopped living by the laws of nature.

Here in the West the industrial revolution, mass manufacturing, modern technology and the establishment of a consumer society have all helped lead us away from a life of harmony with nature. Even more tragic than this is the realisation that we have also lost inner harmony and calm. The various aspects of our personalities seem to be more in conflict than in harmony. If only we could regain what we have let slip away.

Taoists view the world as a holistic unit, that is, it exists as a self-contained organic whole. The same view is held of the Universe, and because mankind exists within this self-contained Universe, he is influenced by it and can influence it in return.

The holistic view is continued in the way that Taoists see the individual. Each person is a combination of body, mind and spirit. An individual's state of health is gauged by how well these various aspects function, both singly and in unity with the other aspects.

It is because of this holistic view that traditional Chinese medicine and exercise therapies, such as acupuncture, herbalism, Dao Yin, Tai Chi and Kung Fu, are as concerned with preventing illness as they are with curing it. Not only do they contain important curative properties, they also provide excellent programmes which assist in establishing and maintaining a balanced state of health for the entire person.

The way of life taught by Chinese martial arts and traditional medicine are all parts of Taoism. Having studied and practised in these fields, I can now see the principal concepts of Taoism working and impacting upon each other in daily life. As a result, I have become more interested in the concepts and philosophy of Taoism. I didn't seek out the philosophy, it found me.

It is not by chance that I happened to write on this topic. I did not set out to write this book, but it did not happen by accident either. This work is a natural progression of my experiences through the martial and healing arts, where I have seen and experienced many of the different aspects of Taoism at work.

As a child my hobby was learning martial arts. As I grew older, the philosophy that formed part of the rich heritage of Chinese culture, healing and martial arts made such an impact on me that I decided to teach my skills and share my experience with others.

The healing aspect of the arts inspired me to study traditional chinese medicine further. It did not take me long to realise that I was skilled and talented as a healer and that I should practise the healing arts on a professional basis. It is in my blood, I have inherited these genes from my forebears. As history repeats itself, here I am doing exactly what members of my family have done in previous generations.

Practical involvement in these various arts helped me understand the Tao more fully. I reached a point where all I wanted to do was to learn more about it, live it and teach it.

During the past twenty years, in which I have lived in a Western culture, I have come to recognise the importance of Taoist principles in daily life. I have seen how Taoism and its healing exercises are of immense value to every individual, from labourers to housewives and executives.

Throughout my career I continued to devote my life to learning and teaching Chinese martial arts and medicine. The next natural step for me was to take out of their theoretical and philosophical contexts the advanced skills I have developed and bring them into the real world. This makes it possible for other people to benefit from them, either through the philosophy or practice of Chinese traditional medicine and martial arts.

In this book as in life, my favourite mind-set, 'The hardest thing is the simplest', is re-lived. In Taoism, Lao Tsu teaches 'work should be done for the joy of it'. That is what I believe. I wrote this book because I could not resist the challenge. I wrote for the value of the work.

The purpose of this book is to teach you the healing secrets of ancient China through the working concepts of Taoist philosophy because the philosophy is the most important tool in achieving health and well-being.

Healing is both a physical and mental exercise. The Chinese consider the mind and the body as one unit. That is why it is crucial to have an appropriate mental attitude in order to maintain or regain health.

You must understand that mental attitude has an important effect upon your health. This is recognised even in the West. The impact of mental and spiritual make-up on physical conditions is well documented in medical literature. An example of this is when people recovering from chemotherapy, as a form of cancer treatment, are encouraged to learn how to meditate.

This book is not a major philosophical work. I will not go into philosophical debates about specific points of Taoist theory. There are any number of worthwhile texts available on a broad range of Taoist subjects. You can refer to the bibliography at the end of this book for further reading.

My intention is to provide you with a practical understanding of Tao and how its beneficial effects can be incorporated into a modern lifestyle. This will provide you with the foundation upon which to build and live your life... in peace, harmony and balance.

We do not have to be sages or hermits in the mountains to practise the principles and enjoy the benefits of Tao. We are fortunate enough to be able to make choices about the way we live. We choose almost everything in our lives, from the food we eat to the hobbies we have.

Choices; that is exactly what this book is about. By acquiring knowledge and skills that can help you take control of your life, you will have an opportunity to improve and enrich your physical, mental and spiritual health.

However, there may still be times in your life when you find it difficult to cope with stressful situations that are detrimental to your health and happiness. It is then that the philosophy of Tao and the gentle healing exercises of Dao Yin will help you the most.

Taoist theory has been taught and practised successfully for over three thousand years. Knowing the basics of Tao theory will enrich your life by allowing you to recognise natural cycles in both your individual existence and the planet upon which you live. If you decide to follow the Tao, you'll find that it is easily incorporated into a modern lifestyle and will provide a refreshing sense of harmony, energy and purpose to your daily life.

In this book, I have chosen to present to you the gentle healing exercises of Dao Yin. It is easy to learn, does not require much time or space, and provides excellent benefits.

Should you prefer to restrict your application of Taoist knowledge to the regular practice of Dao Yin, you will assure your long-term health through these gentle healing exercises which protect you from illness. Dao Yin helps you achieve harmony through the practice of correct breathing, posture, meditation, thought and action. It will allow you to enjoy health and fitness of mind, body, and spirit in a new invigorating and challenging way.

It is your life. It is your choice. I implore you to read on and discover how following Tao can encourage the synergy between your actions and energies to help build an incredibly healthy world for our own and future generations. Experience what it means to be really healthy and at peace with yourself.

Enjoy the book, improve your health and share what you learn with others.

Part I: TAOISM—The basis of the healing arts

Discovering Chinese Taoism

Taoism is the oldest and most popular philosophy in China and it has had an enormous impact on all aspects of life in that country. Its influence can be seen in philosophy, medicine (wholeness, herbalism, acupuncture), art (Yin/ Yang, The Five Elements), architecture (Feng Shui), government (triads, Boxer rebellion), martial arts (Dao Yin, Kung Fu, Tai Chi, Chi Kung), literature and many other aspects of Chinese culture. Without Taoism, Chinese culture would be quite different.

The origins of Taoism lie in the observations of people who were tied to their environment for survival. Through their natural surroundings and the rotation of the seasons they were able to identify their position and purpose in the nature of things.

After centuries of observation, early Taoists came to understand that Taoism is a method of maintaining harmony with both this world and the Universe. It teaches that the actions of Man affect the cosmos (e.g. depletion of the ozone layer) and that Man is affected by the cosmos (e.g. increased infrared radiation, green-house effect).

Tao is often translated as '*the way*' or '*the path*', to Taoists the Tao is '*the eternal ultimate*'. It is both the beginning of all things and the way in which all things pursue their course. It is beyond language and description; however it is not in any sense a creator God.

The Taoists do not conceive Tao as an Omnipotent Being sitting in the clouds. Tao is considered a powerful active force with no human physical representation. Tao creates simply because it is the actual essence of all things. It does not set out to create but things emerge as a result of Tao. It is what the book Tao Te Ching refers to as the 'natural way'.

Tao is the '*way*' or '*method*' of maintaining harmony between mankind, nature and the Universe. It is a holistic system that is not easily accessible from a western reductionist point of view. An indigenous Chinese philosophy, it provides guidelines for living in harmony with ourselves, our environment and universal energies. It is a concept of fitting in with nature, both for our own personal benefit and for the benefit of natural systems. In order to do so we must follow the laws of nature and the Universe.

Taoist philosophy teaches that each part is both a part of the whole and an expression of the whole, that change is the only constant and that everything is relative. There are no absolutes. Nothing can exist on its own. That which exists on a micro level exists and behaves according to the same universal laws as that of the macro level.

Taoism is the concept of yielding or acceptance: Wu-wei (sometimes translated as non-selfishness). It maintains that all things in the universe are created to exist in a state of harmony and balance, and that nature should be allowed to run its course.

Taoism values life, not just human life, but all other kinds of life as well. It is concerned with this life and its perfection with a view to increasing the span and quality of life.

The Tao surrounds everything, every second of the day. It manifests itself in a special kind of energy called 'Chi'. This presence gives life to all existing things and makes possible the 'oneness' that underlies the diversity of the world.

To the Taoists, health is not just the absence of illness. It is a philosophy of life...the way you live your life, your emotions, your thoughts. These shape your health...and your illness.

The philosophy of Taoism gives us the basis to which we should model our life, the basis to which we should live, respond and interact with things around us. Taoism is a way of life that can be lived every second of the day.

Taoism has applications in many aspects of human wellbeing — in the food we choose to eat, in the way we use and manipulate our environment, in our relationships with other individuals, groups and nations, in how we choose to treat illness and resolve problems. To a martial artist, painter, dancer or athlete, it has implications for the very way in which we move.

Taoism is a guide to happiness, peace, self-cultivation, and dealing with the problems of the modern world. Taoists believe that human beings are part of nature and that the key to understanding ourselves and the world we live in, is through increasing our understanding and feeling for others and for nature. By being in harmony with the course of the Universe, we find wholeness, purpose and health.

Tao has always been present in Western and other cultures. Australian Aboriginals do not believe in land ownership. Native North Americans believe that it is their duty to care for the earth and that it cannot be bought or sold. Many indigenous people from around the world have sought to live in harmony with nature since time began.

Let us look at Chinese Taoism through Western eyes.

Taoism through western eyes

'To see a World in a Grain of Sand,
  And a Heaven in a Wild Flower,
Hold Infinity in the palm of your hand,
  And Eternity in an hour.'

William Blake, *Auguries of Innocence*

Eastern philosophy can appear mystical, at times contradictory, to those of us with a western education. But understanding the harmony and balance with nature, the universe, and all things, is basic to the Taoist philosophy.

When Lao Tsu wrote the *Tao Te Ching* in 604 BC, Taoism was already a respected and popular philosophy in China. To put this into perspective, England was still in a state of tribal warfare and the Roman conquest had not yet commenced. Julius Caesar's Roman Legions did not invade Briton until 55 BC., almost five and a half centuries later.

Various people from distinctly different cultures, times and geographic locations relate the same philosophy based upon observations of nature at work. That basic philosophy is the way of Tao, the all-pervasive force that is easily recognised by those attuned to the world of nature.

As a child I would gladly have given any, possibly even all, of my meagre possessions to see just once a living, breathing dragon in all its magnificence, power and glory. How I longed to see the magic in its eyes, feel its hot breath and let its massive strength wash over me. Unfortunately, I have not yet realised that boyhood dream, and probably never will.

However the memory of that burning desire, and the teachings of Tao, make it abundantly clear to me that Taoism applies to all cultures. It is above culture.

We all know that the unnecessary taking of any life is unforgivable. The annihilation of a species, through any but natural circumstances, is positively reprehensible. The hole that the loss of a species leaves in the world which our children will inherit can never be filled.

When an animal dies its spirit is lost from the world. This loss leaves a hole in the fabric of creation and if there are too many holes the fabric disintegrates. Perhaps one way to repair that hole is to encourage another creature of the same species to come into existence.

In modern western language, we talk about any reduction in the planet's biodiversity being an irredeemable loss. We speak of our deep concern that the magnificent animals which share this planet with us will be reduced to museum displays and special-effects movies. We fear that their wonder and splendour will be absent from the lives of our children, replaced by nothing more than myth and memory.

It is of little significance that different cultures, employing a variety of languages, describe the Tao in different ways. That would be a normal expectation regardless of the topic being discussed. More importantly, the very first lines of Lao Tsu's *Tao Te Ching,* are:

'The Tao that can be explained is not the eternal Tao.
The name that can be named is not the eternal name.'

In other words, Tao is beyond description in any language. No matter what lengths we go to in attempting to describe it, it is much more.

Taoism is not foreign to western culture, the concepts are always evident to the careful observer. Universal laws and natural cycles do not stop at immigration to have their passports checked. Many Taoist concepts have crept across our cultural borders and subsequently have been adopted in western literature, music, art and other fields. Such is the power of it's all-pervasiveness.

Even the Bible shows some Taoist tendencies; as in Ecclesiastes 3:

'To everything there is a season, and a time for every purpose under the heaven.'

In our literature revered authors such as Walt Whitman and Henry David Thoreau have described Taoist concepts. This continues to be the case in modern popular literature. Tom Robbins, author of *Still Life With Woodpecker, Even Cowgirls Get The Blues*, and others, writes about many Taoist subjects.

Modern physicists are discovering parallels with ancient Chinese laws. Fritjof Capra in *The Tao of Physics*, comments that eastern mystical ideas fully support his claim that ancient philosophies provide a consistent philosophical foundation for modern scientific theories.

In western art and photography there have been many works, such as those from M. C. Escher, that demonstrate Taoism's dynamic interplay of Yin and Yang.

Western music and poetry contain numerous Taoist references and themes. Many modern day songwriters such as Bob Dylan have written about Taoist concepts. The Desiderata, an anonymous work, is Taoist philosophy even though it was written by someone who in all probability had never heard of the Tao.

In ancient China, physicians were paid as long as their patients remained healthy; and when illness occured, payment stopped. Healing, the Chinese way, is based on the principles of prevention rather than cure. This view has long been shared in the West. Thomas Edison (1847-1931) said "The doctor of the future will give no medicine but will interest his patients in the care of the human frame, on diet, and in the cause and prevention of disease." This is exactly the art and science of traditional chinese medicine.

Modern western medicine is returning to the Taoist concept of treating the whole person and his environment rather than just the individual parts. Here the most important aspect of environment involves family and friends as they have the power to influence the health and recovery of the ill person. Having long ago broken away from the holistic approach, western medicine followed the path of reductionist theory. Establishing and maintaining the health of the entire individual (physical, emotional, mental and spiritual) was replaced with merely treating the symptoms of disease.

Health, to a Taoist, is not just the absence of disease, it is the union of a healthy mind and body which allows us to achieve physical, emotional, psychological and spiritual well being. It provides us with wholeness and purpose by bringing us into harmony with the universe.

However, most of us have never had the basic theory, the pattern of interrelationships and its practical applications to modern life adequately explained. This has made it difficult to observe and benefit from the workings of Tao in every level of daily life. It has also deprived us of a wonderful foundation upon which we can establish the healthiest of lifestyles.

The Chinese proverb: *'See the New in the Old'* comes at an appropriate time for us in the modern world where much help is needed if we are to salvage what we have nearly lost.

So let us look at the essence of Taoist philosophy.

The essence of Taoist philosophy

'All things are One,
    You are part of the Whole,
Belong to It,
    Follow the Natural Way.'

Pier Tsui-Po

In Chapter 32 of the *Tao Te Ching*, Lao Tsu talks of the Tao as being forever indefinable. It is the power beyond power and it flows through the world, like a river heading to the sea, back to its origin.

Man's purpose within this all-encompassing plan is to act as mediator between Heaven and Earth. The price he pays for this privilege is to bear the responsibility of protecting and nurturing all life forms on the planet. To achieve this harmony with nature it is necessary to develop a peaceful mind and spirit in a healthy body. This can only be achieved by living in accordance with the forces of Yin and Yang.

Tao is the ultimate source of all, the origin before origin and the essence which creates everything. The process of eternal creation is told in the following way in Martin Palmer's, *The Elements of Taoism*, where he translates Chapter 42 of *Tao Te Ching* as:

'The Tao is the origin of the One.
The One created the two.
The two formed the three.
From the three came forth all life' (p. 48).

10

The Tao is the origin of the One

The Tao is the ONE. It created itself, simply because the possibility to do so already existed.

Tao moves all things in their essence, but without purpose or intent. This is the concept of non-interference (Wu-wei). The unity of all in the Tao means that in any action that is natural, which occurs rather than is forced, the Tao is active. Putting it in human terms, the Tao Te Ching describes the perfect sage ruler as one who governs in such a way that the people are unaware that he governs them and simply believe that what happens is nature's way.

In acting naturally, by non-interference, by just letting things be and following *the Way*, the sage ruler becomes in harmony with his own essence, the Tao. Being in harmony, he is in unity, and all his actions will thus express this unity and further it. This is the core of the idea that the Tao gives birth to the One.

The One created the Two

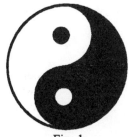

Fig. 1

The Two are the twin forces of Yin and Yang. These forces are complete opposites. Black and white; male and female; hot and cold—they represent within them all that is and can be, but in necessary opposition.

In their eternal struggle, which is the struggle of natural forces not gods, they generate a special kind of energy (Chi) which fuels the creation and which causes all to come to birth. They are not forces of good and evil as they are often presented in the west.

They are locked in an eternal struggle which neither can win. At the very moment that one reaches the highest point of its power it gives way to the other. This is why the Yin/Yang symbol shows the two forces curled around each other, with a dot of the other in the centre of each. All things have their origin in the interaction of the two opposites of Yin and Yang.

The symbol is split into two equal divisions, Yin being represented by the black division and Yang being represented by the white. The small contrasting circles within the larger division represent the fact that within Yin there is Yang and within Yang there is Yin. The dynamic curve represents the continual cyclic struggle between the two forces. Yin and Yang are responsible for the existence of each other. They control each other and transform into each other.

Earlier I mentioned that in order for Man to live in harmony with the Tao it is necessary to live his life in accordance with the forces of Yin and Yang while maintaining an attitude of non-interference or Wu-wei. Here are some examples of how this is achieved.

Examples of living in accordance with the forces of Yin and Yang:
• sleeping (Yin) at night (Yin).
• activity (Yang) during the day (Yang).
• waking with the dawn, resting in the evening.
• warm clothes in winter, cool clothes in summer.
• warm foods in winter, cool foods in summer.
• slow activity in autumn and winter, increased activity in spring and summer.

Comparative Table of Yin and Yang

Yin	Yang
Female	Male
Passive	Active
Night	Day
Soft	Hard
Cold	Hot
Interior	Exterior
Downwards	Upwards
Empty	Full
Contract	Expand

Fig. 2

The Two formed the Three

...From the Three came forth the 10,000 things

The 'Three' is the triad of Heaven, Earth and Man which is the form by which all living things come into actual existence. The link between them is set forth in Chapter 25 of the *Tao Te Ching*:

Tao is powerful;
Heaven is powerful;
Earth is powerful;
Mankind is also powerful.
These are the four great powers of the universe.
And the wise Man takes his place amongst them.

Within the Heaven, Earth and Man trilogy, Heaven (Yang) represents the Spirit or Essence, Earth (Yin) represents the substance and Man, with his feet on the Earth and his head in Heaven, is both the synthesis and mediator between Heaven and Earth. In the human body, this is represented by the energetic mechanism of the 'Three Heaters'.

Man is affected by both the Tao of Heaven and the Tao of Earth. If either one of these is violated, he dies.

The Tao of Man leads us into the areas of the Four Seasons and the Five Elements, which I plan to cover in a later volume.

Branches of Taoism

In ancient times, the main forms of Taoism were contemplative, philosophical, alchemical and physical.

- The *contemplative* form was a meditative observation of the world in which we live. An example of this is the incorporation of animal movements in various exercises.
- The *philosophical* branch dealt with discussion and analysis of Taoist theory. This led to the production of work by authors such as Chuang Tsu and much of the mental skills taught today.
- *Alchemical* was a nature-based art which sought transformation of the physical body through ingestion of various herbs and minerals in an attempt to gain immortality. The modern discipline of Chinese Herbalism evolved from alchemy.
- In the *physical* branch, Taoist exercise programmes aim to improve health and increase longevity through regular maintenance. Based on a balanced diet and special physical exercises such as Dao Yin, Tai Chi, Kung Fu or Chi Kung, attention is given to promoting the internal balance of Yin and Yang and regulating the flow of Chi throughout the body.

You would expect that life in the modern world would be different from ancient times, it is not. We are still human beings, our physiology has not changed, except that we have removed ourselves so far from living a natural lifestyle that we require artificial measures to sustain our life.

Today a combination of these forms of Taoism is practised by those who want to enjoy and benefit from living a natural life. Some of the techniques have been amended and improved to suit our modern physical and mental makeup.

In summary, the main points of Taoist philosophy are:

- everything is part of the whole;
- everything is an expression of the whole;
- everything contains Yin, Yang and Chi;
- the only constant is Change;
- let things occur naturally rather than force them (Wu-wei).

The diagram below shows the relationship between the Tao and everything else, the all-encompassing plan...

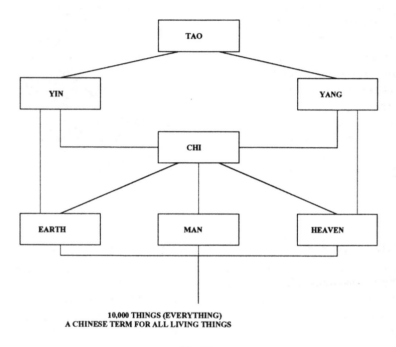

Fig. 3

Let us now look at Yin and Yang, the source of power and the beginning of everything in creation.

Yin and Yang

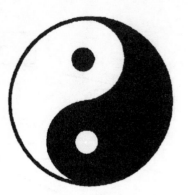

In everything, in every part of the Universe is Yin and Yang.

It is usual for people to see Yin and Yang as positive and negative aspects, but this is basically incomplete, sometimes incorrect. Yin and Yang are natural forces and Taoist philosophy maintains that everything natural serves a positive purpose. Nature is never classified as negative. Yin and Yang are complementary opposites.

The specialised seedpods of many Australian native plants, such as the Banksias, will not release their seeds until they have been subjected to intense heat. This requirement is often met by bush fires sweeping across enormous areas of the landscape. While a raging bush fire causes enormous death and destruction, it also provides myriad opportunities for birth and regrowth. Because of this it can be said to have performed a positive function as well as a negative one.

All actions and applications of force or power result in both Yin and Yang consequences. Even in Western education, Sir Isaac Newton's third law teaches 'For every action there is an equal and opposite reaction'.

You may find it easier to relate to a more three-dimensional example. So let us use the nut and bolt as our example of Yin and Yang working in unison. The bolt (the male component) is Yang, while the nut (the female component) is Yin.

The thread, elements of which are contained in both the Yin and Yang components, represents Chi. We will look at Chi in greater detail in the next chapter. For now, it is enough to realise that it is the thread which allows the nut and bolt to work in unison and provides them with strength. Each component is reliant upon the other two to achieve its purpose.

While most things are broadly segregated into Yin and Yang, it is essential to remember these fundamental principles:

All things contain both Yin and Yang

Here are some examples that illustrate this point:
Time: night and day
Universe: heaven and earth
Seasons: spring and summer (active)
             autumn and winter (inactive)
People: Front of the body is Yin and the back is Yang.

Any Yin or Yang aspect can be infinitely divided into both Yin and Yang aspects

Within any Yin or Yang aspect there is also elements of both Yin and Yang present. For example, hot temperature can be further divided into boiling hot or moderately hot.
Planets in our solar system all rotate around the same sun. Because of their varying degrees of Yin and Yang they are quite different in their physical appearance and makeup. Mercury for example is burning hot, Pluto is freezing cold and Earth is a happy combination. Each planet, whatever its general environment may be, has its warmest (Yang) areas around the equator and its coolest (Yin) at the poles.

Yin and Yang mutually create and transform each other

17

Both Yin and Yang progress through a cycle of transformation from one extreme (hot summer) through a period of moderation (autumn) to the other extreme (cold winter).

They can either transform naturally and in harmony or change suddenly due to disharmony. If you were to run as fast as possible for as long as possible you would eventually collapse from exhaustion. This is an example of excess Yang suddenly changing into Yin.

Yin and Yang control and balance each other

When Yang is too weak, Yin becomes excessive. An illness of heat in the body (fever) may be due to insufficient Yin, likewise penetration of cold in the body (flu) may be due to insufficient Yang.

Yin and Yang are relative

You can distinguish a Yin or a Yang aspect but not separate them. Yin and Yang depend on each other for their definition. For example, to define light, you have to know what dark is. Objects can not be adequately described without using a Yin or Yang aspect. Also, a day or 24 hour period is made up of day time and night time.

All things have their origin in the interaction of Yin and Yang. Complete opposites, these forces represent within them all that is and can be, but in opposition. Life itself is a delicate balance of Yin and Yang. When these forces are properly balanced within us we enjoy a harmony of mind, body and spirit.

The Taoist Yin/Yang symbol provides a visual representation of the basic mechanics of Taoist philosophy. The outer circle is a representation of Tao and symbolises the universe as a whole, self-sufficient unit which contains both Yin and Yang. Consequently, the circle is differentiated into two equal divisions, Yin being represented by the black division and Yang by the white.

Neither Yin nor Yang can ever truly dominate the opposite force, for at the very moment that one reaches the highest point of its power it transforms into the other. This is one reason why the symbol shows the two forces curled around each other, with a small circle of the other in the centre of each. The small contrasting circles enclosed within the larger divisions are also used to illustrate the belief that an element of Yang resides within Yin just as an element of Yin resides within Yang. Nothing is absolutely Yin or Yang.

The dynamic curve which separates these two fundamental elements symbolises both the continual cyclic interplay between the forces and the energy Chi, which is both a product and catalyst of that interplay. Chi, which fuels the creation and causes all to come into existence, is generated in the eternal struggle between these two natural forces.

Like Einstein's theory of relativity, Taoist philosophy maintains that nothing can exist in isolation, that everything is relative and that contrast is essential. This explains why Yin and Yang are considered to be responsible for each other's existence. They control each other and transform into each other. Consequently, any imbalance in either Yin or Yang results in a corresponding imbalance in the other and also interrupts the flow of Chi.

Earlier I mentioned that in order for man to live in harmony with the Tao it is necessary to live in accordance with the forces of Yin and Yang. A few easy ways of doing this are:

- sleeping (Yin) at night (Yin)
- work and exercise (Yang) during the day (Yang)
- arise (Yang) with the dawn (Yang)
- rest (Yin) in the evening (Yin)
- wear warm clothing (Yang) in winter to compensate for the cold (Yin)
- wear cool clothing (Yin) in summer to compensate for the heat (Yang)
- eat warm foods in winter and cool foods in summer
- slow activity in autumn and winter
- increase activity in spring and summer.

It is obvious that no great effort is required to follow this in daily life. You are probably doing so and not aware of it. The Chinese say that if you conciously follow Yin and Yang, you will not get sick.

You may consider that we live the way we do for practical reasons. That is true, to a degree, but it sheds no light on the problem of gradual physical, mental and emotional deterioration experienced by shift workers. The Yin/Yang philosophy quickly and easily provides both the reason for and solution to the problem. A logical, obvious and practical theory which has value, meaning and application in our daily lives, it is used to describe how things function in relation to each other and the Universe.

Yin and Yang fluctuate in cycles that occur both in nature and within the human body. That is, they move from energetically active phases (Yang) to resting phases (Yin). At various times energy must be stored, assimilated and consumed. The early phase of this cycle is when energy is drawn inwards and concentrated (Yin). Once sufficient energy has been accumulated to allow a specific activity to be carried out, the energy is then expended (Yang). For example, one moment the human heart is filling with blood (Yin), the next moment it is forcing blood into the circulatory system (Yang).

Yin and Yang in the human body

Due to its efficacy in treating many conditions without drug related side effects, there is a growing faith in the use of Traditional Chinese Medicine (TCM) throughout the world. However, although it is now widely accepted in Western medicine and recommended by the World Health Organisation (WHO) for the treatment of numerous disorders, the average person has extremely little knowledge of TCM.

TCM is based upon the principles of Taoism. The TCM concept of a healthy body is one in which the Yin and Yang energies are balanced or in harmony. It is a body which continues to function well while experiencing continual fluctuations in the Yin/Yang balance.

The fundamental purpose of the TCM practitioner is to ensure that the patient has an abundant supply of free flowing Chi. This can only be achieved if the Yin and Yang are maintained in a balanced state. Establishing and maintaining a correct Yin/Yang balance enables one to enjoy a harmony of mind, body and spirit.

Illness develops if this harmony is disrupted by an excess or deficiency of either Yin or Yang which fails to correct itself. If either aspect is out of balance it eventually causes disruption in the opposite aspect. Consequently, the production and movement of Chi is impeded.

For example, too much Yang creates heightened organic activity and produces symptoms of dryness, thirst, fever or headache. If you develop a fever, you may become lethargic, agitated, disorientated or even delirious. On the other hand, excess Yin (excess cold) which creates a blockage in the movement of Chi, may result in shivering, joint pain, spasms, or contractions.

Obviously both the physical and mental aspects of our beings are influenced by the forces of Yin and Yang. Our emotions constantly fluctuate between excitement or anger (Yang) and lethargy or sadness (Yin).

As you can see, the interaction of Yin and Yang is a very old philosophy, but is still very relevant today. To understand its full importance we need to look at Chi, which is both the product of and the catalyst in the interaction of Yin and Yang.

Chi—the vital energy that makes life possible

---

*'All things are caught up with yin and carry yang within.
When they combine, then the energy (Ch'i) of life is created'*

Martin Palmer, *The Elements of Taoism, (p. 48)*.
Translating Chapter 42 of the *Tao Te Ching*.

The whole process of life is based on Chi. It is a part of and surrounds everything.

Chi is a combination of Yin and Yang. Everything in the universe (organic and inorganic) is composed of and defined by its Chi. Taoist philosophy considers Chi to be the energy which makes existence and life, in their myriad forms, possible. No English word or phrase can capture its meaning, but 'Chi' is usually translated as 'Vital Energy'. It is more than that. Chi is the vital energy that makes life possible.

Chi is not psychic or paranormal in nature, as was previously believed. It is very real and can be both felt and experienced but not seen. Recent studies have demonstrated that Chi is an actual, empirical energy of extremely high conductivity. However, Chinese thought does not distinguish between matter and energy, so neither classical nor modern texts speculate upon the nature of Chi in any detail. Rather, it is perceived functionally; that is, 'by what it does'.

The all-encompassing universal Chi is subdivided into three major types. In chapter twenty-five of the *Tao Te Ching* Lao Tsu teaches that:

Man obeys the earth.
Earth obeys heaven.
Heaven obeys the Tao.
Tao is the way of Nature.'

The Chi of Heaven, is the Chi of the universe which exists beyond the earth. It controls and co-ordinates the actions of the celestial bodies and has considerable influence upon the Chi of both Heaven and Man. Its influence is carried out through phenomena such as the energy produced by the sun and the gravitational pull of the moon upon the tides. The Chi of Heaven is in turn influenced by both the Chi of Earth and the Chi of Man.

The Chi of Earth is the awesome power of the earth to continually provide life. It absorbs Heaven Chi and is profoundly influenced by it. Even minor fluctuations in the amount of energy received from the sun have dramatic impact upon the earth's climate.

The Chi of Man (humanity) is as individual as our fingerprints. It is our life energy and shapes our personality. We project our Chi into items that we use. For example, when we put someone else's shoes on our feet, even if they are the correct size, they will feel uncomfortable.

The Chi of Man is influenced by, and interacts with, both Heaven Chi and Earth Chi. Mankind, like all living things, relies upon Earth Chi for food and upon Heaven Chi for a habitable climate.

Through its influence upon Heaven Chi and Earth Chi, the Chi of Man provides humanity with the opportunity to live in harmony with the Tao. Unfortunately, in many instances the Chi of Man has had a destructive influence on Heaven Chi and Earth Chi. This is readily apparent to anyone prepared to take a walk along the nearest river bank in a major city. Man's Chi is represented by the degradation of water quality and the refuse lining the bank. The life that once flourished in the river has been destroyed by the Chi of Man.

Your Chi is your physical, mental and spiritual make-up. In other words, your personality and the way you behave.

Chi in the human body

Without Chi life itself would be impossible, because Chi is the 'Vital Energy' or 'Life Force'. Chi has both Yin and Yang aspects which must be balanced and co-ordinated. A smooth distribution of Chi is essential for the body to operate efficiently. This is why Chinese health exercises and medicine concern themselves with maintaining the proper balance of Yin and Yang.

To maintain a strong and healthy body one must learn how to keep Chi circulating smoothly. Daily practice to increase the amount of Chi in the channels and to build up an abundant store of Chi for future use also improves the quality of the Chi. When Chi is abundant within the body one enjoys true health. Disease and depression vanish and longevity is increased.

The Chi within the body, has both substance and function. These aspects are inseparable because each function is based upon a specific substance, just as each substance satisfies a particular function. Food Chi is an example of substance (material Chi), while the channel (meridian) system exemplifies functional Chi.

Chi flows throughout the body via the channel system over a 24 hour period. Channels, a network of pathways that connect internal and external parts of the body, act as a medium through which Chi, blood, and body fluids are distributed. The various types of Chi make use of the channels as their orbit of circulation.

Chi, which is in constant motion, moves in four primary directions: up, down, in and out. So it can be said to ascend, descend, enter or leave. Whenever the movement of Chi ceases the vital functions stop and death ensues.

At various locations along the channels, which run both on the surface and deep inside the body to the organs, are acupuncture points. These points act as safety valves through which the flow of Chi may be regulated. Varying degrees of treatment in regulating the Chi can be obtained by employing either pressure, massage, acupuncture, moxibustion, therapeutic exercises, diet or breathing therapy.

At this point an intelligent person with a reasonable Western education and an average knowledge of human anatomy is probably wondering how such an essential and diverse system can exist within one's own body without our being aware of it. The answer, quite simply, is that there are many things about our own bodies of which we are blissfully unaware until someone else points them out or until something goes wrong.

Types of chi

In general terms, all the Chi in the body is called Normal Chi or True Chi (Zheng Chi or Zhen Chi). This is the name it is given before it is differentiated into specific forms or associated with specific functions.

The Normal Chi is gained from three distinct sources and is a *combination* of: Original Chi/Source Chi (Yuan Chi) which is inherited from our parents, Grain Chi (Gu Chi) is gained through ingesting food, and Air Chi (Kong Chi) is acquired through breathing pure natural air. Normal Chi then permeates throughout the entire body in different forms.

Yuan Chi is the originator of all types of Chi. It is inherited from our parents and is the foundation of Yin and Yang energies in the body. The strength of Yuan Chi determines a person's life span. Its quantity cannot be increased. It is easily depleted. It is related to the reproductive functions, influences growth and development, and it is stored in the Kidneys and Dan Tian.

The mechanism for the production of Chi in the body relies on Original/Source Chi (Yuan Chi) which acts as a catalyst in the formation and transformation of one type of Chi to another. Some of the main types of Chi are:

Zong Chi (Acquired Chi or Clean Chi): This is formed after birth, when we begin eating and breathing, from the essence of food and atmosphere. One of the main functions of Zong Chi is to nourish the heart and lungs. Consequently, it is also called Essential Chi. It gathers around the chest and is concentrated at point Shan Zhong (Conception Vessel 17), meaning 'Sea of Chi', where it influences the relationship between the Heart and Lungs.

Zong Chi aids and regulates movement, respiration and heart beat. It is also related to strength of respiration, voice and movement of blood. It descends from the chest to the Dan Tian, an area the size of your palm located about three centimetres below your navel. The breathing techniques used in Chinese martial arts have been developed to work in conjunction with Zong Chi.

Ying Chi (Nutritive Chi): Ying Chi circulates through the vessels and nourishes the organs. It is the part of Chi which circulates with blood. Its main function is to generate blood fluid and nourish the whole body as it circulates.

Wei Chi (Defensive Chi): Wei Chi is fierce and bold by nature and cannot be controlled by the vessels. As a consequence of this it cannot be contained and circulates outside the vessels. Although it is distributed in the muscles and skin to warm and nourish subcutaneous tissues, its main functions are controlling the opening and closing of skin pores and protecting us from invasion of pathogenic influences such as Wind and Cold. During the day Wei Chi goes to the skin and muscles. At night it withdraws deep inside the body and lies in the chest.

Jing Luo Chi (Meridian Chi): The sensations obtained during acupuncture when working with points on the meridians indicates that the Meridian Chi is exerting its influence and performing its functions.

Organ Chi (Zang Fu Chi): Yuan Chi which circulates in the organs becomes Organ Chi and is named after the particular organ with which it is associated. For example Heart Chi, Lung Chi or Spleen Chi.

The functions of Chi

Chi is very real and alive. It moves and has a purpose to fulfill. The five main functions of Chi are summarised below. They are evident in each of the various types of Chi.

1. Activating Function: Chi is a very strong activating force. The birth and development of the body, together with all its physiological and metabolic activities, rely on the movement of Chi. Chi is the source of all movement and accompanies all movement.

For example, physical activity (walking, dancing), voluntary action (eating, speaking), involuntary movement (breathing, heart beat), mental activity (thinking, dreaming), development, growth and life processes all depend upon the movement of Chi.

2. Protecting / Resisting Function: Chi protects the physical body and resists the penetration of external pathogenic Chi such as Cold or Damp.

3. Transforming Function: Chi is the source of all harmonious transformation within the body. Food is digested and transformed into other substances such as blood, sweat, tears and Chi itself. These changes depend on the transformative function of Chi.

4. Holding Function: Chi governs retention of the body's substances by preventing excessive loss of various fluids such as sweat, saliva and urine. It also holds the organs in their proper place.

5. Warming Function: Chi warms the body and maintains its temperature. Continual fluctuations in the production of heat are required in order to balance the impact of a constantly changing temperature in the external environment.

It is the interacting of all these different types and functions of Chi that produces your physical, emotional, mental and Spiritual state. It is through the manipulation of these forces that traditional Chinese medicine and healing arts bring about their effects.

Now that you understand the fundamental concepts of Chi, Yin and Yang, let us look at how to use your energies—the keys to better health.

Part II: THE MENTAL SKILLS— Establishing well being

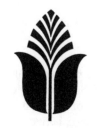

Balancing your energies to prevent disease

'The ancient sages did not treat those who were already ill;
they instructed who were not ill.'

Yellow Emperor's Classic of Internal Medicine,
Translation by Ilza Veith, (p. 53).

Through the powerful force of the Tao that allows life to be possible on planet Earth, every human being at birth inherits a special power that is transformed into various types of energies that the human body uses for the preservation of life.

Ilza Veith in the *Yellow Emperor's Classic of Internal Medicine*, writes:

'Man had received the doctrine of the Tao as a means of maintaining perfect balance and to secure to himself health and long life'. (p. 17).

Only when balance and harmony have been achieved can Man really live with the Tao.

Illness can be prevented by preserving and following the energies of the Tao. To do that, one should follow the way of Yin and Yang, the two dynamic energies which form the basis of health in the body. This energy is needed if you are to be in a state of balance, harmony and health.

It is said that one could live a long life and enjoy constant good health if balance and harmony is achieved. Conversely it would be difficult to live in harmony with the Tao should one suffer from sickness; hence the notion of prevention rather than cure.

Taoism values life. Therefore it is the responsibility of the Taoist to preserve his being and everything else that manifests life, for life is a manifestation of Chi and the interplay of Yin and Yang. So everything that contains Chi and Yin and Yang must be preserved.

This chapter teaches you how to build health. It also makes you more aware of the various causes of illness according to the Taoists. Therefore you'll be in a better position to prevent or resolve illness.

Causes of illness

The Chinese view of health is very different to the western view. Where the west intervenes only when illness is present, the Chinese promote the prevention of disease.

The Chinese way of health is to live in harmony with nature, the seasons and the time of day.

Ilza Veith on page 152 states: *'The Emperor said: Thus life itself is really the beginning of illness.'*

From birth, humans are faced with the reality of having to prepare themselves against the onset of sickness. Without proper knowledge, a whole life can be spent in sickness.

The Taoist view of Tao is seen as the balanced and harmonious way where Heaven, Earth and Man are all seen fitting together as an inseparable whole. When this balance and harmony is separated from the whole, sickness occurs.

The concept of Tao is reflected in the principles of Chinese medicine where balance and harmony are considered to be the fundamental requirements for the existence and maintenance of health. It is regarded with utmost importance that balance and harmony prevail within humans, between humans and society, and between humans and the natural world.

Human sickness is thought to be due to imbalances that result when humans do not live in accordance with the universal laws of nature. Any change in the Yin and Yang harmony alters humanity's physical, mental and spiritual balance.

Causes of human sickness and disharmony are seen in the three areas that reflect the Tao—climatic conditions, emotions and lifestyle.

Not only could these factors affect the health of humans, but it is also known that illness is related to a change in culture or society.

Environment, emotions and lifestyle, on their own or in unity affect our energies.

Any one of our energies, singularly or in combination with each other forms an intricate network of pathologies.

For example, physical, mental and internal energies are affected by our way of life or emotions and the state of the environment affects the quality of external energy, and all the other types of energy as well.

The maintenance of health is vitally important. To prevent illness, you should pay attention to the influential energies that are present in climatic conditions, emotions and way of life.

Disrupted harmonies cause disease; therefore the quest to regain or maintain health is directed towards re-establishing disturbed balances or maintaining current balance and harmony.

Climatic conditions

Humans are affected by climatic factors such as Wind, Cold, Heat, Damp, Dryness and Summer Heat. These are natural events that occur on Earth and can be manifested as pathogens (agents causing disease). They cause sickness if the strength of the body's anti-pathogenic Chi is weak and the body cannot fight off the pathogens, or, if the disease-causing pathogenic Chi is too strong for the body. Excessive exposure to any of these climatic factors lead to disorders in the body.

The climatic factors enter the body from the outside through the mouth, nose and skin to become pernicious energies inside the body. Sickness occur as a result of a losing struggle by the anti-pathogenic Chi against the pathogenic Chi. The body's own Yin and Yang balance becomes affected and an abnormal change develops through either an excess or a deficiency of Yin or Yang. The invasion of the pathogen therefore becomes reflected through the appearance of signs and symptoms, of both the mind and the body.

Once a climatic factor invades the body, sickness is manifested in symptoms or signs that represent that particular climatic factor. As Wind in nature moves the leaves and branches of a tree, Wind inside the body is represented by constant movement such as spasms, convulsions, abnormal movement of the head, limb or trunk. Furthermore, a climatic factor that invades the body could also complicate and lead to many other illnesses. For example, penetration of Damp that accumulates inside the body can eventually give rise to Heat to produce a Damp Heat (combination of damp and heat) pattern of disharmony.

An example of Taoist teachings of life during the spring season reveals that spring is related to the Liver and Gall Bladder organs and marks the beginning of the Chinese New Year. This is the time to start things as Yang is rising. Humans should rise early and exercise gently. The body should be rewarded but not punished with exercises. Wind is the climate of spring and steps should be taken to avoid Wind penetrating the body. If Wind does penetrate the body, it most likely will harm the functions of the Liver.

Emotions

Excessive or insufficient emotions can cause disease.

Humans are able to, where appropriate, experience all the types of emotions such as joy, anger, sadness or grief, pensiveness and fear or fright. The emotions in themselves are not regarded as pathological. Like the climatic factors which are present in the environment, the emotions appear in a healthy and well-balanced person.

Emotions are directly influenced by your physical life, but they also have the power to affect your physical body. For example some forms of stress cause skin conditions such as eczema.

Illness therefore arises when a person is hypersensitive to an emotion, or when a particular emotion becomes either excessive or insufficient over a long period of time. A sudden flare-up of an emotion with great force or a very intensive or persistent emotion that is pent up inside could result in the development of a disharmony, hence sickness. Anger for example, with its effects on the Liver's free flow of Chi and blood could lead to Liver dysfunction. On the other hand a dysfunction of the Liver could lead to sickness that is reflected in emotional behaviour such as easily becoming angry.

A climatic factor such as Cold could also cause emotional disharmony. A person may be severely affected by Cold to an extent that a fear of Cold develops. The disharmony here would not only be in the syndrome of External Cold Penetration but it would also reflect in the function of the Bladder or Kidney (loss of bladder control) as they are related to the emotion of fear.

Lifestyle

Because all living matter (vegetation, animals, humans) is affected and influenced by the Tao, life should be lived in harmony with the Tao in order to avoid illness. One should avoid actions that are contrary to nature so as not to jeopardise balance and harmony. Nature should be left to take its own course as interference could result in sickness.

Diet, sexual and physical activities should be balanced. As the production of Chi and blood is influenced by the food we eat, the energetic qualities of food should be mixed to provide a well-balanced mixture of Yin and Yang types of food. An excessive consumption of Yin (cold, raw) food harms the Yang function in the body such as transforming and transporting the essence from the food. Irregular food intake, voracious eating or insufficient nourishment as well as indulgence in bad food such as fatty food or alcohol eventually lead to sickness.

Physical activity should be regulated as an excess leads to a deficiency of Chi and blood and can cause stagnation of both. On the other hand, a lack of physical exercise leads to stagnation in the flow of Chi and blood throughout the body.

Excess sexual activity is said to not only injure the Kidney but also injure the Heart and the Shen (Spirit) due to their close relationship with the Kidney.

Other miscellaneous factors such as burns, bites, stress, parasites and trauma are also recognised as affecting health.

To summarise, the three major causes of illness are climatic conditions, emotions and lifestyle, so let us see how we can maintain health.

Prevention of illness—building health

As well as receiving the benefits of well-balanced, nutritious food, in order to build health, we also use a synergy of four different types of energies:

- physical (muscular)
- mental   (psychological)
- internal (gift of life)
- external (environmental).

These energies are interdependent. They do not act individually and they are usually harmonised to become one force.

The potentiation of that synergy gives us a power that resides within each one of us, the power to resist climatic pathogens from penetrating or invading our body, the balance within our power to be able to adjust to or accept various degrees of emotions without being affected by them, and the power to cope and recover from the occasional unplanned demands of the stresses of our modern way of life.

Physical energy is obtained through physical activity where muscles are used for movement. This is used in every microsecond of your life, even at rest. Therefore muscular tension affects your physical vitality.

Physical exercise is the best way to cultivate this energy. Activities such as walking, Tai Chi, swimming or Kung Fu helps you develop and strengthen the physical energy required to move your body. These exercises renew the youth of the body by improving the strength, elasticity and flexibility of muscles, ligaments and tendons. Blood flow is improved and the system is purified. That way you can grow old without feeling old.

More common in our modern society is the depletion of mental energy through excess emotions such as worry, anger and fear. The daily tasks of thinking also draw on this reserve.

Mental energy can be regained or recharged. It depends on the state of your physical energy and the amount of mental stimulation you give your mind.

If you are mentally depleted your physical energy level will naturally be the same. Constant learning, improving, discovering and becoming more spiritually conscious recharges mental energy.

When the mind is not calm, peaceful and balanced, the organs cannot function normally.

Internal energy is the part that we are born with. As we start to move in our cot and begin to crawl or walk, we cease to use this energy. At that stage we start to rely on our physical energy which makes our internal energy dormant.

Fighting bacteria in the blood stream is one way our internal energy works for us without our command. It is invisible to the human eye but its effects are visible. You could fall ill if it becomes weak.

Internal energy generates heat. It is stored therefore it can easily be depleted if wasted. This internal energy reserve can be supplemented by food and air Chi.

External energy is the energy that bathes everything in the Universe. This is the most important energy because it is this that brought the universe into being. It created, and made life possible for plants, animals, humans and the whole universe to exist as it is today.

It penetrates humans, plants, animals...everything. It is this energy that descends from heaven, enters into earth to re-energise itself and then goes back to heaven again.

This energy is also good for healing, because the energy that gives us life allows us to give life to others.

The curative properties of herbs, sun and sea are a testimony to the power of external energy. Taking normal precautions, go outdoors, absorb and enjoy it for this is also the gift of life.

It is said that early Taoists lived for over 150 years when they learnt to store and control this energy for their use.

You have now learnt that in order to build health, you need to incorporate all these types of energies into your daily life as well as making adjustments to, or taking precautions against, the elements that cause illness, namely climatic conditions, emotions and lifestyle.

Let's recall the advice given from the *Yellow Emperor's Classic of Internal Medicine* as translated by Ilza Veith:

'There was temperance in eating and drinking. Their hours of rising and retiring were regular and not disorderly and wild. By these means the ancients kept their bodies united with their souls, so as to fulfill their alloted span completely, measuring unto a hundred years before they pased away' (p. 97).

Let us now learn about the part of Taoist philosophy which helps us transform our character and attitudes towards nature and life. It provides us with the opportunities for personal growth and allows us to assist nature to pursue its course.

Self-discovery

'It is much better
To embrace simplicity,
To know one's self,
To reduce selfishness
And moderate desires.'

Tao Te Ching, **Chapter 19.**

You can find the strength within to heal yourself and cope better with the modern world.

You have to get into the habit of doing something to improve your health every day because health is only a habit...lots of small habits that accumulate to give you your desired result.

Unless humans are healthy, nothing else will be healthy. If people don't care for themselves, they will not care about anything else. Think about that.

We have messed up the planet badly for ourselves and for future generations. But, with corrective action by all of us, however small that action might be, we can make life and the world better for every living thing.

To live by the Tao, you the modern Taoist require changes in how you live your life, how you think, how you see yourself and others and how you see the universe as a whole. It is a process of self-improvement that everyone goes through. I have gone through it too and expect to continue to evolve with the change. Some people call change evolution. They resist change but accept evolution. Strange, isn't it?

To live according to the Tao means to adapt oneself to the order of nature and to pursue a way of life in accord with Tao's Ultimate Law.

The various forms of Chinese martial arts for example, through this understanding of nature, made possible certain specialised exercises which mimic the movements of animals such as the horse, crane, snake, among many others. These specialised exercises have developed into the arts we practise today.

Taoists believe that observing nature and its Way (Tao) leads to harmony...and reaching a stage of spontaneity in action that comes from, and with, oneness...in all of nature.

The Tao's Ultimate Law advised us to live in balance and harmony. The following chapters deal with the practical application of achieving that. I have selected some of the main principles of Taoist philosophy that are most appropriate for use in our modern society.

- Yin and Yang and You
- Wu-Wei
- Food as a therapy
- Mother Nature's children
- Inspiration from within
- Taoist exercises for the mind and body
- Self-affirmations

Harmony with these principles must be simple and effortless, otherwise there is no harmony.

Harmony means that you are in unity with all your actions and all your actions express this unity and further it.

Living the Tao on a day-to-day basis will help you to understand more about the Tao instead of merely relying on written or spoken words. You have to experience it with your whole body to appreciate its values. There is no need for questioning or justification of its presence, proof is not necessary.

You must take an active role in both the state of your health and in healing yourself because *your health is your responsibility*. No one else's.

Ultimately the person with the power to heal you is yourself!

So let us explore how you can live your life with the Tao and be the modern Taoist who has the power to heal yourself.

Yin and Yang and you

As discussed earlier, the entire cosmos is held together by the interplay and natural tension created by the positive and negative forces of Yin and Yang. Human beings exist and function in that same way too. All things created become interdependent. Opposites unite as one.

The human body is a link with the harmonious workings of the cosmos. Everyone of us is an element and like the universe, we contain Yin and Yang within. As such, it is subject to all the laws of nature—the ripening and decaying, the heat of the sun to the cold of the winds. Humans and everything else are at the mercy of these cycles controlled by Yin and Yang.

A healthy human body functions naturally on the continual fluctuations between Yin and Yang. Balance and harmony between these two energies are necessary for health and well-being. If this harmony becomes unbalanced, and there is an excess or deficiency of either Yin or Yang that fails to correct itself, then illness develops.

The Moon for example, has long been involved in both earthly and human matters. Ancient peasants have used its cycles to plant their crops by, in order to maximise their yields. Today fishermen depend on the phases of the Moon for tides. Weather forecasters also know that the Moon affects the weather. Ancient medical science has taught us that the Moon affects our health.

There is a link between the phases and position of the Moon and our health. The influence of the energy of the Moon is Yin. This relates to our emotions—moods, feelings and sensitivity. It is associated with very high or very low emotional energy and sometimes erratic behaviours that can go from one extreme to the other.

The state of harmony is a *balance* between Yin and Yang energies where neither one remains at one extreme for an extended period of time. The result of the interplay of these two energies is a number of fluctuations in the balance of Yin and Yang that occurs every second of your day. Only a healthy body can cope with these fluctuations. Chinese martial arts exercises allow the body to regain this much required delicate balance in order that life can be possible.

Here is a set of principles passed on to me by my teachers that will help you finetune your life and achieve greater self-awareness. Take time to fully reflect on them for it is said that those who live by them enjoy increased fulfilment each day.

'He who is gentle (Yin) in appearance but has a strong (Yang) inner character, develops endlessly;
He who is violent (Yang) in appearance and has a stubborn (Yang) inner character, will perish sooner or later.

We are currently seeing the effects of human interference in the natural harmony and balance of Yin and Yang. If continued, that interference will lead to destruction and we will be the first to suffer the consequences, as mentioned in *The Yellow Emperor's Classic of Internal Medicine*, Ilza Veith's translation:

'If, furthermore, the people carefully follow Tao as though it were a law, theirs will be a long life' (p. 109).

The current environmental destruction such as the burning down of the rain forests, extensive logging in old growth forests, drift net fishing, whaling, polluting and many others are all good examples of our disobedience.

The results of this imbalance of Yin and Yang in nature is seen in floods, hurricanes, drought and many other natural disasters. The effects are really much more than that.

Humans are supposed to be caring for the planet, which is a self-perpetuating closed system. If we don't care for the planet then we'll have nowhere to live because our lives are patterned around the natural laws of the universe. We need the sun rays of daylight for growth and repair. We need the regular change and harmony of the seasons to support life. The destruction of this harmony is as disastrous for humans as it is for the entire planet.

People have gone so far from the way it should be. We've got to get back to the beginning.

To live in harmony with Yin and Yang is sleeping at night (Yin) and being active during the day (Yang). Waking with the dawn and resting in the evening, wearing warm clothes in winter, cool clothes in summer, adjusting your diet so that warm foods are eaten in winter, cool foods in summer, slowing your activities in autumn and winter and increasing them in summer and spring.

Yin and Yang are visibly expressed in the cycles of nature. It surrounds us every day. It is usual to see growth or construction, then destruction in harmony together throughout nature. Old trees die and fall to the ground, degenerate and fertilise new trees that strive to reach maturity. The ocean waves build up and then crash on the sand in a release of energy. The year cycles through the seasons.

The hot bright sun creates heat which is Yang. This in turn ascends to heaven, which is therefore considered to be an accumulation of Yang. Yin descends to earth and earth is said to be an accumulation of Yin. Man in the middle is forever subject to the forces of heaven and earth.

Heaven, the Yang element of Tao, can be used to forecast the future global economies. This is because, no matter how technically advanced a society may be, it is still dependent upon the availability of natural products such as food. Detailed scientific analysis could provide valuable information relative to anticipated changes in the natural wealth of various geographical areas. For example, the extended drought in Africa has had a dramatic impact upon their national economies, people, animals, plants and upon the whole environment.

Taoism is living one's life according to the forces of Yin and Yang, the natural way of life. It is living in harmony with nature, finding the path where you merge the forces of Yin and Yang and keep them balanced within the realm of your life. To remain healthy you must attune yourself and your actions to conform with this ever-moving cycle.

With higher consciousness, you can tune yourself to the whole universe. Becoming aware and sensitive to its ever-changing power means that you'll live a healthier and happier life. Start right now.

Wu-wei

'Tao does not strive to achieve,
Yet nothing is left undone.
If mankind observes this,
All things will develop naturally'.

Tao Te Ching, Chapter 37

There are many translations for Wu-wei, such as non-action, non-selfishness or non-interference. In this book I can only explain the meaning to you in words and when you do the Dao Yin exercises described in the latter part of this book, you will experience it for yourself. I have chosen to use the Chinese words for consistency; that way you can form your own opinions regarding how you would like to understand Wu-wei.

As a way of life, Wu-wei is quite simple, tranquil and easy to achieve. It is acting with purpose while avoiding resistance and supremacy or dominance. It is living with a deep inner calm every moment of your day.

This is often misunderstood as being the withdrawal of the Taoist from the wider world with all its temptations and illusions. It was encountered time and time again in the stories of the sages. This technique is the withdrawal of the Taoist from the false path which the material world is taking. It would be a great mistake to think that is all there is to Wu-wei.

Wu-wei is most often translated as *non-action*. This is not meant literally as 'inactivity', 'doing nothing', or 'withdrawing', but rather, '*taking no action that is contrary to nature*', that is, letting nature take its own course without being destructive.

Non-action has been interpreted as completely withdrawing from participation, which can mean that you let others make decisions that affect you. That is not how I learnt the Way of the Tao.

It means not to dominate and to let others have their say and contribute. Once this is applied, true synergy can both be witnessed and achieved. This is what the Chinese call 'action without action'.

This is not to say that Taoism is excessively passive, for example, nature can be violent with earthquakes and cyclones. These natural acts can occur quite quickly, with or without warning.

Taoism is not a philosophy of infinite quietism or withdrawal. It is a philosphy of non-interference, and that is what I prefer to call Wu-wei: 'non-interference'. The *Tao Te Ching* teaches Wu-wei, but also gives practical methods for action.

Non-interference means that you take an active interest that is quiet, not over-bearing, while achieving harmonious results for all, man and nature. It has been my experience that quietism is incredibly powerful. It cannot be seen but can only be experienced.

It means giving others a chance to contribute and getting the best out of them. Things are achieved because you go with the flow or way of the Tao, rather than interfering and forcing events to occur. It is the willingness to let go. However there could be circumstances where both extremes need to be balanced in a harmonious way.

The concept of Wu-wei indicates that one should avoid planning and striving that is contrary to the flow of Chi, but observe and move carefully with the flow of compatible opportunities as they arise.

My personal experience of Wu-wei is that it has been designed to assist us in discovering ways of being true to ourselves, to help us associate with other human beings, the physical world and the universe around us.

All actions result in both Yin and Yang consequences, so it is better to make many small changes than a few major ones. This minimises the unfavourable aspects and allows other natural systems to adapt to our behaviour.

My grandmother used to tell me, 'Take care of the small things and the big things will take care of themselves.'

One of my favourite sayings is 'Don't push the river', meaning 'don't force what is already a natural flow'. This is appropriate in matters regarding life and existence.

This principle forms the basis of the teachings of Chinese martial arts and is often illustrated in the way true masters teach their pupils. Pupils are not harassed into learning at a rate that satisfies the master. They are educated at whatever rate they are best able to cope with the physical, mental and spiritual development. It can be very harmful to push the pupils or teach them higher skills before they are ready to embrace them.

The key to Lao Tsu's system is Wu-wei—'doing by not doing'. According to his ideas, man should be still and passive before the workings of nature, of Tao, the 'right way'.

Taoism is the concept of yielding or acceptance, Wu-wei. It maintains that all things in the universe are created to exist in a state of harmony and that nature should be allowed to run its course.

Wu-wei is the art of being in such harmony with the universe that everything happens as it should, as though it is meant to be. It just happens.

Let us now look at therapy by food...

Food as therapy

'If an illness is to be treated, treat it with diet therapy first, then with drugs if it is not cured.'

Sun Si Miao (581-673 AD), *Thousand Golden Prescriptions for Emergencies.*

Life force energy (Chi) is received from food which provides one of the three sources of Chi in the body. Therefore it needs to receive your special attention.

Traditional cultures use food for medicine and nourishment. Some foods are also used as symbols to represent certain aspects of their culture.

Food has a nutritional and a healing (remedial) property. Given the absence of disease, nutrition is received through regular sustenance on a daily basis. The healing property is the balancing or resolving of acute or chronic conditions as well as a therapy to prevent illness. Today, this is left mainly in the hands of Chinese herbal medicine practitioners.

Basic nutritional foods are both practical and inexpensive. Unlike most forms of medication, they can be used forever without harmful side-effects.

A properly balanced diet based on the principles of traditional Chinese medicine helps create internal balance and harmony, whereas improper diet is a direct cause of ill-health.

Diet-related illnesses of the past such as scurvy, gout or goitre are not common today but modern conditions such as heart disease, gastrointestinal disturbances such as bowel cancer and others can still be relieved or prevented by proper nutrition. Psychological illness such as anorexia nervosa and schizophrenia can respond well to dietary improvements.

49

Food as a therapy is used in Chinese medicine today.

Food is selected for its energy, flavour and *movement of its Chi*. How it affects meridians, organs, bodily functions and symptoms are also important. Contra indications for the use of some foods are also offered to ensure that food is selected for the proper condition or illness.

For example, cucumber has a cool and sweet energy. It detoxifies, promotes urination and quenches thirst. It is also effective in relieving acne. This is because acne is due to excessive heat in the Lung and Stomach Chi. This is balanced by the cool energy of fresh cucumber. The Chinese preserve cucumbers and eat them as a vegetable to cleanse the blood, clear up internal heat or relieve hot skin conditions. The juice of a squeezed cucumber can be applied externally to affected areas to relieve burns. The leaf of the cucumber plant is also effective. Even old cucumbers that have turned yellow are used. They are boiled as a soup to ease dry cough in the autumn as the season exerts its pathogenic energy of dryness. The symptom of coughing is because the lungs are most susceptible to external pathogenic influences.

Unlike the ancient alchemists, today we do not ingest gold or mercury to prolong life. Gold is still used today in the treatment of arthritis. We have learnt about the toxic effects of mercury, which is fatal to humans, animal and plant life, yet for the past 150 years we have continued to allow dentists to use mercury (amalgam) in our tooth fillings.

Your health depends on the goodness and quantity of the food you eat. Correct eating and drinking habits will change your life. You'll feel much healthier and have more energy. Your eyes will sparkle, your skin will glow, your attitude will be more positive, your vitality will be infectious and your brain will not let you down. You will sleep better and your outlook on life will be optimistic.

Our ancestors ate natural grain foods, vegetables, fruit and herbs that were not tampered with by Man. Today the focus on food and eating is rarely for nourishment. Instead it is used for celebration or just to fill a hole and usually on the run, not realising that this contributes to a short, unhappy and unhealthy life. With decoration, colouring and preservatives, food is made more attractive but it is not always fit for your consumption.

The Chinese believe that there is a direct relationship between the quality of your life and the quality of food you eat. You can achieve balance and improve health through good selection, preparation and serving methods, regular eating times, methods, conditions and frequency. Eating imported foods out of season, upsets the balance of Chi in your body.

The natural produce of the current season is most likely to be right for a balanced diet at that time of year. For example, temperature is a very important aspect of a balanced diet. Hot or warm foods (Yang) heat you up and cold or cool foods (Yin) cool you down. This is why we eat hot soups in winter and salads in summer. The vegetables in the soup are grown and available during winter months and the salad foods grow in the summer months. In winter, one should eat food with warm or hot energy such as ginger, ginseng, leek or walnut. The hot summer months are soothed with food which has a cool or cold energy such as barley, bean curd, cucumber, eggplant or grapefruit.

The Tao teaches us to avoid extremes and keep an overall balance. With food from every part of the world available all year round, the balance is easily upset. Taoists maintain that food eaten should be from the same geographical region. If you are in the winter season, you should eat winter produce and not the summer produce which is readily imported from another part of the world.

Recently, western society has changed its attitudes towards diet. Many people now advocate the need for more organically grown fruit, vegetables and cereal fibre accompanied by a reduction in meat and animal fats, refined foods, sugar and salt. This is along the lines of a Taoist diet.

Taoist philosophy advises *balance*. Due to the ancient Taoists' natural way of life and high respect for animal life, they were mainly vegetarians. Today not all practising Taoists are vegetarians but this does not mean they do not have respect for animal life. There are many issues, values and situations and debating these is beyond the scope of this book. The decision as to whether you choose to be a complete vegetarian or considerably reduce your intake of animal flesh is beyond this book. Meanwhile, I recommend that you reduce meat intake if you have not already done so and eat more grains, fruits and vegetables.

It is important to point out here that I have found that in the preparation of oriental herbal remedies, there are quite a number of plant substitutes for animal parts that are equally as effective and do not require any animal, endangered or otherwise, to bear or suffer from cruelty of any kind.

As far as is known, the practice of using animal parts in the preparation of herbal medicines is endemic. I believe that in the future many more practitioners of traditional Chinese medicine will also substitute equivalents.

As a child in the countryside I vividly remember seeing on many occasions members of my family killing animals for food. It was a very distressing event but the taking of that life was done in a very honourable and respectful way. Words cannot describe what I saw. The animal was taken only when there was a real need. Only the quantity needed was taken. That is, a chicken would be used instead of a cow. There was no waste. First the taker would place himself before God and then he would ask the animal for forgiveness, for the act that was about to occur was a necessity for survival, not greed.

Here are some basic principles you can follow that will enormously improve your health:

- Eat only when hungry and do not over eat. Try to eat three to four small meals a day on a regular basis.
- Eat only natural foods. (Avoid processed, synthetic or chemically enhanced foods.)
- Eat more natural whole grains, vegetables and fruit in season. Choose organically grown food.
- Chew your food to a paste.
- Drink pure water or herb teas.
- Avoid animal fat. Reduce meat consumption to a healthy minimum.
- Breathe clean air often.
- Avoid cold food and drink if possible; room temperature is best.

In the *Synopsis of the Golden Chamber*, Zhang Zhong Jing, a distinguished physician of the Eastern Han Dynasty writes:

> '...food and drink are beneficial to health, but only when taken
> appropriately both as to quality and quantity; otherwise, they

can become detrimental. Moreover, for sick persons, suitable food will be beneficial to the recovery from illness, while unsuitable food aggravates the condition.'

To help our body assimilate the nutritious and remedial aspects of food, we need to take time out to experience being ...

Mother Nature's children

'The universe has a sacred spirit.
You must not interfere with it.
Trying to improve it, you will ruin it.
Trying to hold it, you will lose it.

Tao Te Ching, Chapter 29.

The essence of Taoism is the belief that human beings are just one very delicate part of the whole picture. Humanity is considered to be a minuscule part of nature, and the key to understanding ourselves and the world we live in is through the understanding of nature.

Taoism holds that as long as humans are in harmony with nature, they will flourish. If nature is contravened and disobeyed, the individual suffers through physical or emotional illness.

It also taught that life should be lived in harmony with the Cosmos, the seasons, the time of day and with one's own constitution and stage in life. For example, physical, mental and internal energies are affected by our lifestyle and its consequent emotions. The state of the environment affects the quality of not only External energy, but all the other types of energy as well.

Tao relates to many aspects of life. It teaches you that every single area of life is connected, not just mental and physical health, but the condition of your vital organs, your feelings and emotions, behaviour, your diet, how and when you eat your food, your breathing, and your spiritual life. It also relates to how you respond to your surroundings, such as other people, animals, soil, ocean, environment—the whole universe.

We seem to function separately from everything else when in actual fact we live in a totality, in a sea of energy, where everything is totally interconnected.

This principle is evident in everyday life. Looking at our planet it is clear that we are part of an interdependent system. The smallest things have significant effects on us and our surroundings. Bacteria can kill us, yet those which are in a symbiotic relationship with us, dwelling in our gut, are also vital to the function of processing food.

Over the years we have seen many examples of the complex consequences of our interference with ecosystems; how the introduction of an insect or animal can have drastic unforeseen effects.

In Taoism, the world is seen as a holistic unit. Man affects the Cosmos and is affected by it. Taoism as a philosophy leads to the development of actions which are methods of maintaining harmony with this world and the Universe.

Practising Chinese martial arts is a way of moving straight to an intuitive way of understanding Taoism, bypassing the words and intellectualisation of philosophical discussion.

A key element of the understanding of the Tao or the 'Way' of the Universe through martial arts, is that all things are connected to each other. Tai Chi and Kung Fu, for example, aim to harness this fundamental interconnectedness. In both of these arts, the practitioner is taught to perceive the slightest shift of weight on the foot which precedes a sudden attack, like the spider which can perceive the faintest movement in its web, no matter how far away. Such is the power of Taoism in action.

Tao teaches us to be very cautious and respectful towards nature and to recognise that we are part of something much greater and more significant than we can possibly imagine. Tao ensures people follow the way of nature (natural laws) and abide by its powers and rights.

The law of Tao explains that everything you do affect the entire world, and that likewise everything that happens in the world affects you. We can change the world simply by changing ourselves first.

I believe the future of our planet depends on how we look after ourselves. First we need to truly value our body and soul. Then we will be able to protect and conserve nature and allow the environment to survive. After all, the environment, which is an organ, breathes and needs clean air like we do. It depends on clean rain for water like we do and survives on its own clean waste just as we survive on the uncontaminated food it provides us.

So start living the Tao right away. You will become physically healthier and internally and mentally stronger. You will then discover the other dimensions of the universe. As you progress though life, you will start to notice things that you have not noticed before.

Here is a technique I learnt years ago that I recommend you do every day. It is a simple meditation, awareness and self-discovery exercise that is easily adapted to your daily life.

Stop for just one minute every hour.

In that hour, look, think, feel and experience life in the incredible universe that you are part of.

Because you only get one chance at life.

Inspiration from within

'The sage knows himself but does not boast
He loves himself but is not vain
He rejects "This" to choose "That"'.

Tao Te Ching, Chapter 72

From the very beginning Taoism taught that the way you behave, think and feel, change your physical and mental well-being, your health.

Change

A rolling stone gathers no moss. The Tao Te Ching teaches that change is the only constant in the Universe; it happens unconciously and naturally in all things and in all circumstances.

Poet and musician, Bob Dylan sang *'The times they are a-changin'*. That was in the early 1960. Today, thirty years later, there is a global movement for change and improvement, yet many are still resisting, gathering moss.

Life is about transformation and change. Nothing stays the same. We change. Situations change. Our perceptions change. Life changes...so accept it.

But is change the way to keep up with change? The opposite appears to be also true because in essence, people are still the same. Henry David Thoreau said that *'Things do not change; we change'*.

Some of us think that change is insecurity or chaos. There is a tendency to feel the need to impose some order and therefore resist or control change.

Usually we feel safer and more comfortable in our own world where nothing changes and everything is predictable. Life is not like that. The Tao is definitely not like that either.

To make your life more focused and enjoyable, requires some change on your part. Assess all the dissatisfying parts of your life and make it better. To be a better person requires you to be a different person. The greater the effort you put in, the greater your reward. For things to get better, first you have to be a better person.

Taoism teaches that change is the only constant. It is both inevitable and irreversible. Nothing remains the same unless it has chosen to die. In everyday life you can see the perpetual change of the seasons, the varying degrees of light between sunrise and sunset. Look at the plants in your garden and you will quickly understand why change needs to be constant and why it is an essential aspect of harmony and balance.

Change itself continually creates opportunities, and for those who stop to recognise its importance, change can be an advantage.

So what stops us from truly changing for the better?

Paradigms

Our willingness to change is affected by our paradigms, that is, the way we see the world. We do not see the world the way it is, we see it the way we expect it to appear, as we are conditioned to see it. Paradigms govern the way we see things and the way we see things governs how we behave.

So for us to really see things the way they are, we need to change our paradigms; because the future outcome of our life depends on what is within us. Our inner spirituality provides us with our first source of inspiration. Inspiration from inside keeps us on the right track. Balance and harmony come through accepting and moving with change. That way you can see life as it really is, because clarity is power.

Co-operation with the ways of nature leads to harmony with nature, while disregard for the ways of nature leads to disaster.

To accept and evolve with change, the Tao teaches that everyone has a purpose in life, the reason for one's existence on earth. In many cases it has already been planned for us, and it is unchangeable.

Purpose—the direction in your life

In the very last lines of the Tao Te Ching, Lao Tsu writes that the more one does for others, the more he has; and the more he gives to others, the greater his abundance. To be effective in 'doing for others' or 'giving to others', we need to live our lives with a purpose.

Throughout my growing-up years, I noticed that quite a few of my teachers would regularly provoke me to think about a question that would eventually shape my life. Each asked in his own way but essentially it was this same question: *'Tell me Pier, what is your purpose in life?'* At that time I hated hearing the question and it did not make any sense, until one day the meaning came to me.

They taught me that purpose should be never-ending, and that I should make it my passion in life. Purpose is not to be confused with goals. Goals are small achievable results whereas purpose gives direction in your life.

Purpose is a spiritual thing. It is your core, your personal mission. Not everyone readily knows or can identify their true purpose. You can discover your true propose if you live according to the Tao, become more spiritually conscious and more in touch with your inner self. It will take time to find this answer.

In a lifetime, people usually have a few insights into what they think is their purpose, only to learn later (often through financial or personal setbacks) that what they had chosen to do was not their true purpose or direction. I have personally experienced many of these *learning experiences* (mistakes) myself.

It can come to you any time, anywhere or in your dreams. You will know by the quality of ideas and by the feelings these ideas produce, like a 'this is it' feeling. Just trust your intuitive intelligence.

Your subconscious mind is the place of wisdom, knowledge and power to guide and instruct you. It has the answer, and by going deep within yourself you are able to reach the source of information in your subconscious mind that is not usually accessible to you under normal circumstances.

Doing what you are supposed to be doing does not mean doing what you love doing. I love being in the sun on a tropical island, but that is not what I am meant to do in order to contribute to the welfare of this planet. My purpose is to help people heal themselves but I will not achieve that by swimming in the warm waters of the tropics.

In finding your true purpose you may have a few setbacks, so you need to learn from these experiences and persevere until you find your true purpose or direction.

To succeed, you need to be fully committed, which means *never going back*. And when you do decide to fully commit yourself, ask yourself these questions:

- Who and what will I have helped?
- What will I have learnt in the process?

My teacher once told me it is said that these two questions are asked when one leaves physical life.

Do what you can, because without healthy people and a healthy planet we will not survive. Special talents are not required if your purpose is to serve others, for the betterment of all lifeforms and our planet.

Also ask yourself these questions:

Are you proud of what humans have done to this planet?
Are you proud of what humans do to animals, plants, other people?
Are you proud of what people do to themselves?

60

Are you proud of what you are doing to yourself?

If not, you can do something about it right now.

Here is an easy start. Relax, calm yourself fully and just take a minute to yourself and write down *one single thing you can start to do right now that would make a positive difference to your personal life*. You can repeat this same question if you need to improve your health, finances, career, or relationships.

To the Chinese this is the very first step towards the journey of a thousand miles.

Once you have decided on that 'one thing', the key is to continue with it every day. Try it. The results you would get from the synergy of just that one little thing will amaze you. Just for a moment, imagine the difference.

No one can alter the path that has been spiritually laid down for you. They say that the Tao will guide you. Resisting the inevitable leads to imbalance of Yin and Yang, therefore illness or unhappiness occurs. So go with the flow and give your inner being a chance to recognise opportunities—for that is living the Tao.

The Ancients say that if you do what you are supposed to do, you will be rewarded in many ways: health, happiness, finances and in many other ways.

Positive Thoughts

Buddha said; *'All that you are is the result of what you have thought, with your thoughts you make your world'*.

Positive thoughts can empower you and others. Refuse to participate in anything negative. Be an optimist.

Your brain does what you tell it to do. Everything that happens to you starts with a thought. All your reactions and behaviours are thoughts. Your past, present or future is a thought. You can change your body with one thought. Any negative thoughts that your brain receives such as those from yourself, from radio and television programmes, from books, newspapers or magazines, from conversations with other people and so on, will eventually affect you.

Sometimes we cannot help being exposed to negative circumstances. For example the media has to report violence for us to become aware of it. Therefore we must know how to react to the news. Your reality is the reality you create. Nothing has any meaning except the meaning you give it.

There is a direct relationship between emotion and thought. Thoughts can make you feel sad or happy or angry and we know that emotions are a key factor in causing illness. So control your thoughts and emotions. Never let a bad thought enter your mind.

Is it scarcity, or is it waste.

I have met many private and business people who have been greatly affected by a deep-seated attitude of 'scarcity', that is, there is not enough to go around for everybody. This is a very damaging negative attitude to take. It creates greed, winners and losers...where some people win at the expense of others. There is no need for this, there is plenty for everyone.

There are many more opportunities in life than any one person can handle. They become scarce only because of our lack of knowledge or action.

Many people think there is not enough to go around. Scarcity exists in people's minds. With food for example, there is little scarcity, if any at all. We are producing much more than could feed the world. We waste so much food in the home and in restaurants. We overeat...much more than our body can cope with. This damages our digestive system and in turn we become diseased.

The problem is also with the distribution of food. The citizens of some parts of Africa or the Middle East will testify to that. Often it is not the people but the system that needs overhauling, where some people continue to cause misery to others.

Live by the Tao

Like others before you who have chosen to live by the Tao, you will need self-discipline at first until it becomes a natural way of life for you. It is a good process to go through and you will not regret it because it will teach you a lot about yourself. Just listen to your body and you will know.

Once you start to live the Tao, go step by step, in easy stages for it cannot be hurried. Everything happens in stages. They say that you will only see when you are ready to see or only hear when you are ready to hear. So go easy on yourself. Then learn to preserve and accept it, like you accept the wind that blows, the spring that follows winter and the day after night.

Remember that you only need to change your ways just a tiny bit at a time. That small change you make today will synergise into quite an enormous difference over a period of time. Imagine this example from aviation where a half-degree shift from the flight plan means that the aeroplane can be one hundred or more miles off course.

We need to bring back and re-experience the values of respect, love, trust, integrity, happiness, truth, justice, patience and caring to our modern world if we are going to survive as humans.

For our planet to survive we need to have courage to think and move sideways to do what has not been done before, despite criticisms of being different, so that we can stop doing what we have been doing for far too long...destroying, plundering and exploiting.

To live with the Tao calls for courage, study, contemplation, daily practice, failure and above all, trying again.

You have the power in you. Do it!

Taoist exercises for the mind and body

'The softest thing in the universe
Overcomes the hardest thing in the universe.
When there is no room for action
Know the advantage of non-action'.

Tao Te Ching, Chapter 43

The body cannot be cured without the Spirit, our core.

We have learnt from the ancient Taoist sages that we must actively participate in breathing, meditation and specific physical exercises to achieve health and long life. The food we eat is also vitally important.

In the west, exercise methods such as walking or swimming develop the physical body and external physical strength. Therefore that places some limits on the benefits of exercise to the *whole* body. Muscular energy is limited to one's strength and endurance, whereas there is no limit to Spiritual energy. The power of this form of energy increases with practice and does so without limit.

Due to the damaging effects on the body, western scientists are currently advising people against strenuous physical exercise such as excessive running or sports.

The method of the Tao develops the whole person: the mind, the inner body, the external body and the spirit. Its exercises were developed to enable the body to exercise in a balanced way. That is, they are neither too physically damaging nor too physically inactive.

The end result of Taoist exercises is to transform you to a state of being calm, quiet and centred, so that you are then able to accomplish your daily tasks effortlessly. Lao Tsu's philosophy teaches that:

- Softness conquers hardness.
- Quietness allows you to listen and understand your opponent's energy or force as we do in martial arts.
- Gentleness develops strength.
- Slow movement hides potential energy, and can be devastating to your opponent.

The concept of living in harmony with the Tao has played an important part, for without this philosophy, Chinese exercise systems, arts, culture or medicine would not have had the essence of being Chinese.

In the *Yellow Emperor's Classic of Internal Medicine*, many references stress that health and longevity depend largely upon your behaviour towards the Tao. Page 100 of Veith's translation tells:

> *'Ch'i Po answered: Those who follow the Tao, the Right Way,*
> *can escape old age and keep their body in perfect condition.*
> *Although they are old in years they are still able to produce*
> *offspring.'*

I believe that 'The real doctor is the doctor within'. So here are two techniques, Positive imagery and joy, laughter and smile, that you can use quickly and easily to help heal yourself:

Positive imagery—creating the right pictures in your mind

What you believe will happen has a powerful effect on what eventually does happen to you. So you need to remind yourself that your body naturally heals and repairs itself. To do that you simply insert thoughts of health and strength in your mind. That way you encourage them to happen.

On the other hand, if you fear disease, you will more likely get the disease because your body feels and responds to the effect of what is thought. The messages you send to your brain master the way your physical body operates.

If you send positive thoughts such as strength to your brain your body will respond to your call and fight off illness or infection. Conversely if you send negative messages like feeling ill, you will no doubt get a corresponding response from your body.

I write my daily affirmations (vows). I do the same for my objectives and purpose, such as 'My body heals itself' on one side of 7x12 centimetre cards that I carry around with me. Each time I have a spare moment to reflect or contemplate, I review my cards. Sometimes I have gone through this process at least ten times in one day. It has benefited me greatly. You can do the same too.

I also use these cards in my daily 'creating' period, the very first ten minutes of every morning of every day. I review my cards at that time. This helps me detach from any negatives that could arise during the day and also helps me re-programme my mind so that I can reinforce my vision, understanding and commitment.

Here is a quick two-minute exercise that you can do at least once every day (or more often if you can arrange the time) to help you heal yourself.

First achieve this easy mental and physical relaxation exercise:

- sit or lie down
- feel every muscle in your body relax, starting with the largest muscles first
- clear your mind, relax the muscles in your face to a point where you feel a gentle inner smile being shown on your face
- feel your mind relaxed
- focus on expanding your belly when you breathe in (called Dan Tian breathing).

CARE: You must be absolutely relaxed and calm both in body and in mind before you continue.

66

Then:

- bathe yourself in thoughts of health and strength
- send these thoughts to every cell of your entire body
- imagine the vital energy (Chi) flowing throughout your entire body
- feel and experience your body as a miraculous healing machine
- acknowledge that you have achieved that state and...
- claim it.

Joy, laughter and smile

Include much joy, laughter and smiling in your life. They do heal. Laughter releases an important type of hormone in the brain—endorphin, which relieves pain, tension and depression.

Research has shown that stressful mental states such as anxiety, worry, fear or greed can hinder your immune system, making you prone to become ill.

These harmful mental states can easily be overcome with the positive imagery exercise explained above as well as including much joy and laughter in your life.

There is an ancient Taoist meditation technique that even allows you to send the feelings of a 'smile' to your vital organs. Imagine how healthy your physiology would be if all these organs were in a 'smiling' mode rather than a 'frowning-unhappy' mode.

Smile and the world smiles with you, how true this is.

Another important technique is...

Self-affirmations

'*Let him step to the music which he hears, however measured or far away.*'

Henry David Thoreau, *Walden, (p. 184).*

A technique that is used to integrate and unify mind and body is the recitation of self-affirmations or 'vows'. It will bring your body to its full power and will focus your mind on your intention.

The recitation confirms one's purpose. It can also be done before, and in some cases, after an activity.

To help you 'keep on the right track' for the day, you can start the morning with a recitation of your vows. This can be done either formally such as during meditation or exercise, or informally such as while shaving or dressing up for work. I prefer to commence my day with a review of my vows each morning while shaving. I have a copy of my 7x12 centimetre 'Morning Card' stuck on the wall of my bathroom for easy reference.

Before a meal, a vow is a way of expressing gratitude and appreciation for the nourishment which our body is about to receive. That moment taken helps us to erase all negative feelings and thoughts and prepare our body to place itself in the most appropriate state so that we can benefit from the nourishment the food provides. In my clinic, it is one of the techniques that has worked successfully in the treatment of obesity. It has helped change people's attitude towards excessive eating by increasing their respect and appreciation for food. The technique voluntarily elevate one's body to a state of harmony, balance and peace.

Vows can be in many forms. Chanting the OM sound (annunciated AUM) is a purifying exercise which stimulates the mind and body through vibration. The OM sound is the most ancient universal sound. Instead, you can choose words that you can recite easily.

In some traditional exercise programmes such as Kung Fu, prior to commencement of the exercise, a vow is recited. This establishes a harmonious relationship between you and the exercises. This can be in form of words chosen for a specific purpose such as to heal a certain illness or to improve an aspect of your life.

In Dao Yin, this practising formula is recited at the start of the exercise. It reminds the practitioner of the techniques.

'Throw away your troubles in the stillness of the night
Thought on Dan Tian
Seal the orifices
Breathe gently
Connect the magpie bridge
Light as a swallow flying in the sky'.

You can write your own vows. Just make sure that they do not contain any negative words or implications. It is best to keep the words simple and not too long. An example of a vow can be

' Everyday in every way I'm getting healthier'.

The vows can be in a form of continuous meditation during your waking hours. It can be repeated at any time. However it is best to repeat or reflect on your vows when your body is calm and you are mentally quiet.

Your self-affirmation cards are the foundation for setting up your proper mind-set. Henry David Thoreau's *Walden*, tells:

'If one advances confidently in the direction of his dreams, and
endeavours to live the life that he has imagined, he will meet
with a success unimagined in common hours. He will put some

things behind, will pass an invisible boundary; new, universal, and more liberal laws will begin to establish themselves around and within him; or the old laws be expanded, and interpreted in his favour in a more liberal sense, and he will live with the license of a higher order of beings. In proportion as he simplifies his life, the laws of the universe will appear less complex, and solitude will not be solitude, nor poverty poverty, nor weakness weakness. If you have built castles in the air, your work need not be lost; that is where they should be. Now put the foundations under them.' (p. 183).

Give it a go and write some of your affirmations. Write one for the morning and one for the evening. Your goals and purpose should be written up also. Any other reminders such as behavioural or attitude changes can also be done in the same way. Try it...and you will not ever regret doing it.

Part III: THE PHYSICAL SKILLS— Taoism in action

The heart of Chinese martial arts

'Succeed,
Because it is unavoidable.
But real success,
Is not gained through force.'

Tao Te Ching, Chapter 30

The true essence of Chinese martial arts is self-preservation and healing. Their official beginning is said to have started when the three sets of exercises 'Eighteen Hands of Lo-Han', 'Marrow Washing' and 'Muscle Change Classic' were introduced to the Shaolin temple in China by Bodhidharma (Buddha). But there were earlier forms of exercise such as those for stretching muscles and others to prevent or resolve the penetration of wind, cold and damp from the environment.

About 300 years before Bodhidharma arrived at the Shaolin temple, Hua To, an eminent Chinese physician who developped the use of anesthetics, was one of the first advocates of preventative medicine. To avoid or curtail illness, he created a series of exercises which he called 'Five Animals Play'. They were created from his observations of the tiger, deer, bear, ape, and bird. These exercises were preliminary initiators of later forms of martial arts which are based on these animal movements.

These exercises have been a continuous part of Chinese culture since earliest days. This meant that when the Lo-Han breathing exercises were introduced they were readily and easily accepted. Eventually the ancient art of Dao Yin developed.

Because of the concepts of Taoism, the ancient Taoists considered themselves to be part of the world. Through studying animals and their natural behaviour, they realised that physical activity is an essential part of daily life. It was also through the understanding of nature that exercises which mimic the movements of animals such as the horse, tiger, crane and others were developed into the arts we practise today.

The basic stretching and breathing exercises were gradually developed and their practitioners eventually formed into three factions. The object of exercise in these factions was either physical, mental or a combination of both.

This led to the development of the internal and external schools. The internal schools concentrated on the development of Chi through meditation and gentle, calming, physical exercise. The external schools were more concerned with physical prowess, believing that it is essential to defend life and health, and to produce powerful Chi.

The internal arts developed into Chi Kung and Tai Chi. The more physically oriented art developed into Kung Fu. The basic theory of all these arts is the same, all Taoist theory. The applications are very similar in their movements because they all developed from the same core.

For example, Dao Yin's 'push the boat downstream' technique is very similar to Tai Chi's 'close the door'. In Chi Kung it is used as a Chi building exercise. In Kung Fu it is a double palm strike in dragon stance.

So, the core was there, and out of that core grew ancient Dao Yin. Out of ancient Dao Yin grew mind and body exercises such as Kung Fu, Tai Chi, modern Dao Yin and other arts.

It is not by accident that the martial arts have always been referred to as self defence arts. The philosophy behind the whole thing is to use the skills to improve the world. No true martial artist would use those skills to take advantage of weaker people. Preying on weakness is both cowardly and contrary to Taoism, as Taoism recognises that weakness is an essential part of the world.

Through learning martial arts people become more aware of themselves.

They gain a higher level of physical control through which they gain a better understanding of their body and mind. Consequently, they have a greater understanding of illness or injury when it occurs. Martial arts training attunes them physically to the philosophy of traditional Chinese medicine. Properly taught martial arts teaches you to have better control over your mind and body.

The more you know about your body and the more sensitive you are to the way it changes or reacts, the better you can keep it healthy. For example, when you go to the doctor with a problem, the more you know and can tell him about your condition the better equipped he is to help. For balance, all the different martial arts have their own Yin and Yang component. If you are currently practising martial arts and don't have that in your classes find a more capable teacher.

Kung Fu, considered a Yang art, is visually very Yang yet there is also a blend of Yin moves in it. Tai Chi and Dao Yin are more gentle therefore considered Yin.

The progress of one's participation in the various Chinese martial arts is intended to reflect that of our own human growth pattern. When we are very young and physically tender we should practise Dao Yin in order to develop a strong, healthy body. When we have the physical capacity required to engage in Kung Fu, we can transfer to that art in order to develop further both physically and spiritually.

As we grow older, the gentle movements of Tai Chi becomes more suitable. While it helps maintain our improved flexibility, balance and coordination, it does not require the vigorous physical effort we were prepared to make in our youth. At this stage of our training it is more appropriate to concentrate on internal power rather than physical force.

In the final stages of our training we can progress further with the internal arts or even return to Dao Yin. Hence the complete circle.

In western society today the selection of an art to practice is a matter of personal preference. Today people have more energies to burn and are more conscious about self-defence and physical fitness, so they are more attracted to

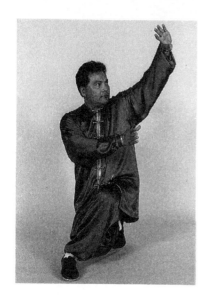

Master Pier Tsui-Po in Dao Yin's 'Push the window open to look at the moon'

Fig. 4

Master Charles Tsui-Po in Tai Chi's 'Holding the ball'

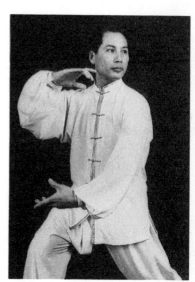

Fig. 5

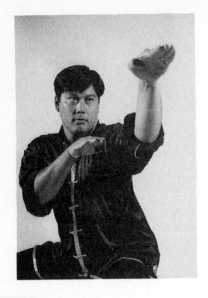

Master Richard Tsui-Po in Kung Fu's 'Snake coming out of the hole'

Fig. 6

Master Steeve Kiat in Kung Fu's 'Eagle Claw'

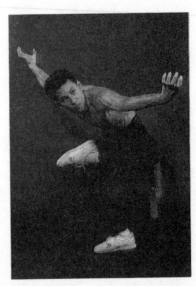

Fig. 7

the hard Kung Fu. Others with injuries or limited abilities find the gentle Tai Chi and Dao Yin more suitable.

The best way to ensure that maximum benefits are gained from the study of Chinese martial arts is by completing the full circle. The beauty of the system is that you can enter the circle at any time and any place. It is never too late. Start now.

Dao Yin healing exercises—how they work

For the purposes of this book, I have chosen to present to you the gentle healing exercises of Dao Yin rather than another technique of Chinese martial arts. Dao Yin is a health exercise programme that is very different to others. It is the art of the future.

Many sources say that the ancient form of Dao Yin is the foundation of many types of Chinese martial arts and callisthenics. It originated over 3000 years ago and it was used to ward off illnesses caused by climate and environment such as wind, cold and damp. The main purpose was to cure and prevent illness and improve health. The exercises consisted of movements learned by watching animals. When the techniques were practised, they expelled the 'bad Chi' that invaded the body to cause illness. That rebalanced the system.

The old techniques have been revised and updated to create the modern Dao Yin. Much of this work is attributed to Professor Zhang Guang-de of the Peoples' Republic of China. In 1976 he started this research after falling ill with terminal disease. He applied his work to his illness with amazing success. He was completely cured of all illnesses and now devotes much of his time to the continued research and development of Dao Yin.

I remember when I was a child at Kung Fu training, the preparatory exercises for the more rigourous part of training were the ancient Dao Yin exercises. Not many of us took notice of its healing properties. We just wanted to get on with Kung Fu. Our teachers used to say that we needed Dao Yin to protect ourselves and not get hurt. We said: 'that is what the Kung Fu is for'.

78

Well I have discovered more than 30 years later that what they really meant was that the Dao Yin is to prevent us from getting sick.

The principles of modern Dao Yin by Professor Zhang are based on the concepts of Chinese medicine, western medicine, Tai Chi and Chi Kung. This system has been honoured by the Chinese people as a 'life-saving exercise'.

Dao Yin combines all the beneficial aspects of meditation, breathing, Tai Chi, Chi Kung and Chinese medicine so that the three levels of body, mind and breath-energy are involved.

There are many different sets of exercises. Each set of exercises specifically deals with one of the systems of the body such as the heart, lungs, liver, digestive and musculo-skeletal system. Dao Yin works by encouraging the cultivation of smooth flow of Chi throughout the body and to specific parts of the body, while also improving the quality of Chi in the body so that illness is prevented or cured.

Each set of exercises is designed to specifically give a healing effect to the body. For example, the set 'Heart function and blood circulation skill' is designed to prevent and cure diseases of the cardiovascular system while the set 'Musculo-skeletal skill' prevents and cures diseases affecting the muscles, bones and tendons.

The exercises are composed of gentle, flowing movements similar to those performed in Tai Chi, so you will not pound or strain your body. They are easy to learn and practise and they are graceful and relaxing. They are arranged into short, easily remembered sets. You only need a short period of time and a small place to practise Dao Yin.

By improving the functioning of the internal organs and systems of your body, Dao Yin assists in resolving and preventing health problems such as stress, fatigue, arthritis, anxiety, digestive disorders, heart and lung conditions.

Dao Yin improves circulation, mental relaxation, concentration and alertness. It increases physical flexibility, strengthens muscles and mobilises the limbs and joints. It helps you to regain your power which is lost during illness or injury.

Proven results and recent achievements

According to Professor Zhang Guang-de, Dao Yin has been applied to clinical use in China with an astounding success rate of 90 per cent. It has been recognised, approved and praised several times by scholars and experts in the fields of medicine, physiology and physical education both in China and abroad.

The exercises to 'Prevent and cure heart and blood diseases' won first prize in the Scientific Research Conference of major institutes of physical education of China, Germany and Japan. It was also listed as 'the national significant achievement in science and technology'.

In the 11th Asian Games Scientific Congress, the exercises to 'Prevent and cure difficult and complicated diseases' was selected as the 'excellent paper'.

Improve yourself and avoid illness

Many people of all ages have recovered from illness and acquired new life or have become healthier and prevented illness by practising Dao Yin. Dao Yin will benefit you by providing you with the much needed balance of Yin and Yang that can improve your health, and prevent illness and injury.

Dao Yin is suitable for people of all ages and levels of physical fitness so that they can work toward their own good health. It especially provides a comprehensive new discipline for the elderly, the middle-aged and for people with certain illnesses to assist in regaining their health and fitness. You will protect and improve your health with Dao Yin.

While the Chinese people practised the ancient Dao Yin for illness prevention, the Taoist masters also used various types of breathing and meditation techniques to achieve supernatural powers. They discovered that life can be lengthened and diseases can be resisted and overcome. They found that illness was caused by an unbalanced flow of Chi, mental and emotional excesses, weakness or deficiency in the level of Chi and external attacks such as by wind, cold or damp from the environment.

As time went by and as life changed, Chinese medical doctors observed that meditation to regulate the body, mind and breathing was not enough to cure and prevent illness. The purity of life since the Taoist sages had changed considerably.

They learned through generations of clinical practice and observation that people who exercised with *specific body movements* to adjust the Chi got sick less often and their bodies degenerated less quickly than others who did not do the exercises.

So a new theory on the cure of illness was born.

The Chinese medical doctors learnt that to increase the circulation of Chi, one must also physically move their bodies. Although a calm and peaceful mind that is experienced in meditation and breathing is important for health, exercising the body was found to be more important and appropriate for the current times.

Unlike other forms of martial arts and exercise programmes, Dao Yin is very different. It emphasises soft, gentle healing techniques that have been specially designed to target various organs and systems. This builds up Chi internally.

Dao Yin exercises improve the quality of your Chi, and stimulate and increase its circulation. This removes stagnation and blockages and lets your body's own natural healing mechanism operate. This is the basis of health and healing shared by traditional Chinese medicine.

The modern Dao Yin is closely integrated with the practice of traditional Chinese medicine. In China, it is taught in hospitals, rehabilitation centres, and universities as part of a holistic approach to the prevention and treatment of illness.

The theory of Dao Yin is profound, therefore the challenge is more significant.

When you do the Dao Yin exercises, your body is involved in a continuous combination of:

- breathing
- meditation, and
- specific physical movements that self-massage and activate various meridians and points on the body.

The meridians are a network of pathways that carry Chi and blood to various parts of the body. The meridians and points used are the same ones used in the science of traditional Chinese medicine such as acupuncture. The points are life-giving, life-regulating and life-support centres in the body that make our bodily functions possible.

When Chi flows through the meridians harmoniously, clearing obstructions and nourishing organs, good health results.

Effects of Dao Yin exercises on your body

The physical movements in Dao Yin involve special ways of turning, twisting and resting weight on some parts of your body. This activates special meridians and points in order to promote healing and prevent illness.

The physical exercises in Dao Yin involve massaging internal organs, muscles and ligaments with specific movements.

One of the theories of Chinese medical acupuncture teaches that the major joints of the body such as the wrist, elbows, shoulders, neck, waist, knees, ankles have a number of major control points that completely surround them. The flow of Chi to your body from these points in your joints is very critical in determining your overall health.

The points influence the flow of Chi to such a degree that they determine the amount and rhythm of the flow of Chi to meridians; hence, to the body parts that follow their path. Therefore a stagnation or obstruction in the flow of Chi through one of your main joints ultimately causes a condition in that joint as well as other minor conditions or illnesses further down the meridian, body part or even in its corresponding internal organ as meridians connect the internal body to the external.

Here are just *two vital points* that are used *throughout* DaoYin's exercises. Other vital points are explained later in the book.

During Dao Yin, the wrist is rotated to a 180 degree angle or more to activate all the major points on the wrist. Specifically the wrist movement activates two of the major points that are critical to the proper functioning of two major systems in your body—the heart and lungs.

These two vital points are: Lung 9 (Tai Yuan) and Heart 7 (Shen Men). They involve the physical, mental and spiritual aspects of the body.

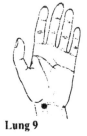

Lung 9

Fig. 8

Lung 9 (Tai Yuan), called 'Supreme Abyss', refers to Chi entering deeply into the interior. It is the Earth, Yuan and Shu point of the Lung meridian. In traditional acupuncture science, Earth, Yuan or Shu points have major significance. It is an influential point of the pulse (arteries and veins). It regulates and strengthens the lungs and its functions. It removes and prevents the formation of phlegm and mucus in the lungs.

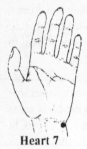

Heart 7 (Shen Men), is called the 'Door of the Spirit'. The Spirit (Shen) is directly affected at this point. In Taoism, it also refers to the eyes, the place where the spirit enters and leaves. Through the eyes one can tell the presence and strength of the Spirit.It is the Earth, Yuan and Shu point of the Heart meridian. It is the major point for the Spirit and helps prevent psychological disorders or emotional instability while helping to harmonise the functions of the mind.

Heart 7

Fig. 9

Most acupuncture points have one major feature. These two points have more than three features. That is why they are so important.

Dao Yin speeds up healing, maintains health and cures sickness. It encourages the reproduction and growth of healthy tissues. Here's how your body responds to the Dao Yin exercises.

1. Promotes a smooth circulation of Chi in the meridians which in turn distributes Chi to both the external and internal parts of your body. This smooth flow will prevent stagnation, obstruction or lack of Chi from occurring in the body, hence allowing the proper functioning of all your bodily systems. Regular practice will maintain a smooth flow of Chi to the entire body so that any damage done can be repaired and strength rebuilt. The health of internal organs can be rebuilt with good flow of Chi and gentle massage actions that take place during the exercise.

2. Slows down the aging process.

3. Strengthens immune and hormone production systems. Our immune system helps us fight diseases. It is also related to the endocrine glands which produce hormones. Hormones in turn contribute to the fundamental processes of life such as growth and reproduction. They can actually speed them up or slow them down.

4. Raises vitality.

5. Gentle exercise benefits your muscles, ligaments and bones. It increases the

strength and flexibility of your muscles which is lost during periods of inactivity or illness. Your endurance level will improve. The weight-bearing exercises increase the strength of your bones. The involvement of your muscles ensures the distribution and return of blood back to your heart for re-oxygenation by your lungs. It nourishes the tissues with good circulation of blood. Your body will be more relaxed and you'll regain your power.

6. Better physical and mental relaxation.

Being calm allows you to be in touch with your inner self. It also removes physical and mental tension and helps alleviate stress, which has been recognised as a major cause of illness in our modern society.

When you practise regularly, your mind will gradually become calm and peaceful so you'll be able to relax and enjoy your daily work and life.

Your whole being will start to feel more balanced, you'll discover your inner world and you'll have more control. Through internal sensing and feeling and examining your inner experiences, you'll start to understand yourself physically and mentally.

Let us now take a look at the synergistic effects of the Dao Yin healing exercises on your body.

Synergistic effects of Dao Yin

There are three levels of achievement: novice, intermediate and advanced. Each level reflects a different level of practice. So it is important that you know what you are aiming for.

The *novice student* aims to regulate the body until he feels relaxed and comfortable. Then he goes on to regulate the breathing and the mind.

Once the physical movements are learnt and can be performed without having to think about them, *intermediate level* students concentrate on using the mind to lead Chi to the points. This ensures the flow of Chi through all the channels. It will help to equalise the balance of Yin and Yang in the body as well as clearing blockages or obstructions caused by emotions or pathological Chi in the body.

Finally, after diligent practice, the *advanced student* learns to regulate the Spirit while using the combination of the previous two levels. The focus is on achieving the ultimate unity and harmony of the mind, body and spirit.

The amount of time required to progress from novice to advanced level depends on each individual. Some need less time than others. Like most other forms of activity, the key to achievement is regular practice, patience, perseverance and inner awareness.

Key to receiving the benefits of Dao Yin during practice

Behind every movement is the whole philosophy of the Tao. The key to receiving the benefits of Dao Yin is to:

* regulate the body
* regulate the breathing
* regulate the mind,

in all movements at all times.

Once this is achieved, you can progress to higher levels by:

* regulating the flow of Chi through the meridians and
* regulating the Spirit.

These last two methods are advanced, but achievable.

Regulating your body

Be fully relaxed

Every cell in your body should be fully relaxed. Adjust your body until you experience deep calmness, feel centred and balanced.

The level of relaxation should go deep to reach the marrow in your bones. That way the Chi can be led from the surface of the skin to deep inside your body to reach the furthest point.

Outward strength or force in movements are not used. This does not mean that you start to slouch, become passive or lose control over your composure. It means that your body is carefully balanced to the point where it is just between passive and active so that your body can be mobilised immediately to a Yin or Yang extreme. A good example of that is the ballet dancer or the non-Taoist swatting of a mosquito.

Keep your body upright and movements coordinated with your waist. This technique will enable your whole body to move smoothly and continuously as one unit.

Be light, agile and natural

Your whole body and your outer movements should be light, agile and natural while your mind reaches for inner sensitivity. That way you'll reduce force or muscular tension.

Slow and continuous movements

The exercises should not be rushed. At first you may need to force giving yourself some time. So take your time, you have got all the time in the world.

Slow movements allow you to relax, become gentle and give you time to concentrate and feel every detail.

It allows you to develop an acute sense of balance while you become more aware of every part of your entire body and mind. It also calms the outside and peacefully benefits the inside, thoughts and emotions.

This is one of the techniques used by ancient sages to experience the flow of Chi throughout the body. It eventually led to the discovery of the channel system that is used in traditional Chinese medicine today. The sages were able to become so quiet that they were able to hear their body at work. You too can do this.

Circular movements

Each movement should have an arc or circle. You may enlarge or reduce the arc or circle to the limit as long as you maintain proper postures.

The Chinese believe that circles generate more force than straight lines. This can be seen in nature for example, when cyclones or tornadoes cause more destruction than the wind that blows in a straight line.

Constant rate

The beginning to the end of every movement is even. Move like the movement of the sun from the time it rises to the time it sets. Jerky or irregular flow of movement imbalances Yin and Yang and disrupts the smooth flow of Chi, which is so crucial to your overall health.

Regulating your breathing

Air is one of the three sources of Chi in the body.

The purpose of breathing during Dao Yin is to build up your Chi to a higher level, both in quantity and quality, in order to protect and strengthen your body.

Two techniques can be used:

- normal abdominal breathing
- reverse abdominal breathing.

In this Dao Yin routine you will only use the normal abdominal breathing; that is your abdomen expands when you breathe inwards. This is called Dan Tian breathing.

Practise this method of breathing until it becomes natural. That was the way we breathed when we were born. Unfortunately, as we grow older and become more tense and stressed, our breathing becomes shallow and is taken over by the chest.

This method of deep breathing will help you to relax physically and mentally and allow the Chi to circulate in all channels.

In Dao Yin, the point Hui Yin (located near the anus) is contracted at the start of each breath and relaxed when breathing out.

Breathing will regulate the Chi flow inside your body. It will make Chi circulate smoothly and strongly throughout the body.

Allow your Chi to reach your skin and marrow and feel it arriving there. This will keep the skin fresh and young and allow the blood manufacturing process in the marrow to function optimally.

Let the Chi flow to your head. This will nourish your brain. As it is the master and controller of your whole being, when it is healthy and functioning well, your spirit and vitality can be raised.

Regulating your mind

The purpose is to become calm and concentrated without disturbance. Then you can use your concentrated mind to lead the Chi to circulate in a smooth way. When your mind is strong, Chi is strong.

When a person's mind is not calm, balanced and peaceful the organs do not function properly, for example depression or anxiety can cause stomach ulcers, indigestion or nausea.

First clear your mind of all thoughts.

Develop your mind, then go on to develop calmness. When you become calm, the flow of thoughts and emotions slows down and you feel mentally and emotionally neutral.

Once your body reaches this relaxed state, your Chi will naturally flow smoothly and strongly. That way you will be able to concentrate and not be disturbed by other things.

Bring your mind to the attention of your whole body, inside and outside. This enables you to feel the Chi circulate in your body.

Once you have developed the ability to readily become calm and quiet, you will be able to balance your thoughts and emotions at any time.

You will also be able to reach into the state of 'transparency' where you can clearly feel the state of your body's Yin and Yang at work. This enables you to adjust your Yin and Yang levels. With years of practice and dedication, Masters of the art have used this technique to reach this state of 'Wu Chi'.

It is said that once you are able to reach 'Wu Chi', you have the power to return your whole Spirit to its origin - that is, the state before your birth. Your Chi and Spirit will then unite with the Chi and Spirit of nature and you finally become one with nature. This state is also called the final enlightenment or Bhuddahood.

Regulating Chi in your meridians

This technique is quite advanced.

It is obvious that in order to regulate your Chi, you need to have a sufficient amount of Chi in your body; otherwise you risk becoming very weak and fall ill. If you feel you do not have enough Chi to do this technique, then work on building up your Chi first.

First, you need to be able to feel and experience the movement of Chi from the previous three techniques described. Then relax your body from the outside skin to deep inside to reach the internal organs and bone marrow. That will also help you to feel and sense your centre.

Lead your Chi to the skin to increase its sensitivity. Follow by sending it to your muscles. Kung Fu training emphasises this technique to energise the muscles and to increase physical power. Then you can try sending the Chi to the bones to nourish the marrow. Once you can do this, you can then try to regulate it by making it flow through the meridians.

If all of this is achieved, you will know that your Chi has been lifted to a higher level.

Regulating your Spirit

To the Chinese, the Spirit originates from the mind and resides in the Heart.

A high Spirit is required in order to prevent or cure illness or create health. This is easily achieved by first knowing why you are doing the exercises, how to do them and what you can expect to gain from them. Part II of this book will help.

To achieve a high Spirit, you need to consider the three fundamental Spiritual roots which are self-explanatory;

- will
- patience
- endurance.

When the Spirit is high the Chi becomes strong and can be directed easily. When the Chi is strong, the Spirit also become strong.

General tips for practice

Every single aspect of Dao Yin benefits the body in a special way. This means that you can select just one part of the exercise when you need it the most. For example, you can do the breathing technique before an interview or to help you cope with a difficult situation.

One way to do this is to ask yourself what aspects of Dao Yin you need most and why you need them. That will help you to select the particular exercise.

It is also important to understand everything behind what you are practising and not just automatically repeat all the moves . Take time to become interested in why and how it works because getting good results means you will need to do the exercises the authentic way. Any deviation in the techniques will not give you the desired results.

Ask yourself what you wish to achieve and what you expect to achieve in doing the exercises. Once that is clearly in your mind you will be able to focus and achieve that goal because if you know your goals your mind will be firm and steady and you will stay focused.

Regularly assess your progress. You will be much kinder to yourself if you know that your efforts have not been wasted. Discovering how much you have progressed will be a great joy and satisfaction. That will help you to improve and advance in the future.

Practise regularly and perform the techniques correctly, because every movement has its special meaning, purpose, way and effect on your body. Use this book and other materials such as tapes. Practise with patience and perseverance. That will help you develop a strong will and lots of self-discipline. Ultimately, you will find peace, quietness and the natural state.

Let us now look at breathing, meditation and relaxation in more detail.

Breathing

Correct breathing is the basis of all exercises recommended in China for longevity as well as for the cure of several diseases.

The philosopher Chuang Tsu promulgated the idea that men of great wisdom fetch their breath from deep inside and below while ordinary men breathe with the chest alone.

How you breathe tells you how you feel about yourself and how you relate to your outside environment.

Breathing is related to emotions and emotions affect your breathing. They prevent equal inhaling and exhaling, therefore the full benefit of breathing is not received. For example, when you are angry or stressed your breathing is short and fast and you exhale more strongly than you inhale. When you are sad you tend to breathe more and when you are excited you exhale longer.

Effects of Dao Yin breathing

Dao Yin breathing relaxes and calms you. It keeps your mind clear and calm. It purifies and revitalises your body.

Correct breathing fills your lungs with fresh oxygen, thereby increasing oxygen supply to red blood cells. Your blood, brain, and every cell in your entire body receives more and fresher oxygen. It helps to cleanse the blood and the body of their debris.

While moving the diaphragm up and down, breathing also massages and stimulates the internal organs.

94

Deep breathing exercises charge the Kidneys with vital energy. Chinese medical physiology teaches that human potential lies with the Kidneys, the body's vital energy storage tanks.

Long, deep breathing releases carbon dioxide which is a waste product that changes to carbonic acid if not removed. Extra carbonic acid is filtered by your kidneys thereby decreasing you body's vital energy.

The main purpose of the breathing exercises is to adjust the balance of Yin and Yang. Taoist philosophy teaches that the action of inhaling allows the Chi of Heaven (Yang) to descend and the action of exhaling allows the Chi of Earth (Yin) to rise. Therefore breathing at the Dan Tian connects these two Chi (Yin and Yang) and also connects and combines humans with Heaven and Earth.

How to breathe in Dao Yin

In Dao Yin you will use a specialised Taoist breathing technique where you take eight Yin breaths and eight Yang breaths.

First try to make your breathing soft, slow, continuous and uniform, even if your inhaling is relatively short and your inhaling and exhaling rhythm is not balanced.

Inhale and exhale to about 75 percent capacity. This will prevent tension occurring in muscles which can also lead to tension in the Mind and other parts of the body.

As you become more experienced, you then aim to breathe longer, deeper, softer breaths. Maintain the continuity and uniformity in your breathing patterns. Ultimately this breathing method will happen naturally, unconsciously.

The next step is to focus your mind on the points and areas which will move and lead the Chi along the meridians to its destination. For example focus on the point Pericardium 8 (Lao Gong) in the middle of your palm. The Chi then becomes activated to move along the pericardium meridian and activates influence on the areas it is responsible for.

Once you become advanced, you will be able to move your Chi to any place you like at will. You will feel, experience and direct your Chi along the meridians to any part of your body.

Ancient Chinese masters also taught that your Chi is where your mind is and that your mind leads the Chi and makes it move. If your mind stops in any one spot, your Chi becomes stagnant. Likewise if you try too hard and become tense your Chi becomes stiff which is what you want to avoid. You want a smooth flow of Chi throughout your body.

As you breathe deeply you will experience a state of meditation, so let us look at meditation.

Meditation

Once you reach the calm, peaceful, meditative state you will release all your mental, physical and emotional stress and tension.

Meditation allows you to break out from your limitations and lets you expand to higher levels of awareness. Each person has different abilities and goes to a different level; therefore one cannot describe the vastness that can be experienced.

Physical power can be increased while quietness and stillness that slows down your metabolism can be achieved. Consequently, the strong powerful Chi in the body can be used to make living easier while the calmness has great therapeutic benefits such as reducing blood pressure, stress or headaches.

During meditation, thoughts will come and go. Let your thoughts go and come back to meditation. *It is this letting go process that benefits the brain.*

The sages say that answers to questions often come through the act of meditation. They say that we have the answer to any question we have and all we have to do is to go deep inside and search for it.

I for one will vouch for this. My wealth of ideas and solutions to situations have always come to me during or after meditation. You will experience the same. I know of many people who use this technique quite successfully in both business and health problems.

Meditation in Dao Yin involves both meditation while being still (still meditation) and meditation while moving from one technique to another (moving meditation).

In still meditation, your physical body should be very still, relaxed, calm. This opens the Chi channels and allows your mind to lead the Chi.

A method of still meditation that you will learn later in this book is called 'holding the moon'. This exercise strengthens the mind and builds up your Chi to a higher level.

To increase the quantity and quality of Chi stored, meditation allows Chi to circulate and build up in the twelve primary meridians while filling up the Conception Vessel (Yin) and Governor Vessel (Yang) meridians. Both these two meridians are major controlling reservoirs of Chi in the body and they are the masters of Yin and Yang Chi respectively. When Chi in these two meridians is abundant, the Chi in the remaining meridians will in turn be abundant; therefore the body is able to function more efficiently and prevent illness.

Every movement used in Dao Yin incorporates the moving meditation. In other forms of meditation, a mantra is chanted. In the Chinese healing arts, *the movements are the mantra*. The breathing performed during meditation also includes various therapeutic sounds that correspond to certain organs and meridians. A healthy organ vibrates at a special frequency in order to maintain the optimal functioning of that organ by preventing or relieving illness. For example the sound wooooo (like blowing out a candle) benefits the Kidneys.

Overall, meditation leads you into the domain of emptiness where your whole being transforms into the 'no extremity' (Wu Chi) state. Once you have reached this, Chi in your body and Chi in nature will unite and become one.

I invite you to meditate regularly because you will not know the beauty of the scenery unless you go there.

To be in the correct mode for meditation, you need to be fully relaxed in both mind and body, so let us briefly look at inner calm, the true relaxation, where a technique that you can use is explained.

Inner calm—true relaxation

You will get in touch with your inner self when your whole being is calm, relaxed, centered and quiet.

All the meridians in your body become open when you are fully relaxed. When the meridians are open Chi and blood will travel freely and blockages can be cleared.

To achieve this, your mind must first be relaxed and calm. When your mind coordinates with your breathing, your body is then able to relax to its deepest level.

There are three levels of relaxation to the physical body;

- postural relaxation
- relaxation of muscles and tendons
- relaxation of internal organs and bone marrow.

To achieve *postural relaxation*, your body needs to be in a very comfortable and relaxed state. Your body must be centred and balanced. This is easily experienced when sitting in a comfortable armchair for example.

It is said that when your posture is not correct, your Chi will not be smooth. If your Chi is not smooth then your mind will not be peaceful. When the mind is not peaceful, then the flow of Chi becomes unsmoothed. This eventually leads to illness.

For better postural relaxation, balance the body and the Heart because the Heart houses the Spirit (Shen). This is done by first relaxing and regulating your mind because relaxation of your body originates with the state of your mind.

Then you go on to place your mind *deep into the muscles and tendons*. Feel every one of their fibres. Start from the head and go right through to your toes. Let the tension out of them.

Relaxation of internal organs and bone marrow is the stage where you can feel transparent, as if your whole body has disappeared. Once you can do that, you can lead your Chi to a diseased organ and cure it. You will also be able to protect your organs and slow down their degeneration.

A simple technique for mind and body relaxation

- Sit or lie down.
- Feel every muscle in your body relax, starting with the largest muscles first.
- Clear your mind, relax the muscles in your face to a point where you feel a gentle inner smile being shown on your face.
- Feel your mind relaxed.

Focus on deep abdominal Dan Tian breathing.

- Let your body relax.
- Feel the calm that goes with it.
- Feel the calm in every cell of your body and your mind.
- Let yourself go.

CARE: You must be absolutely relaxed and calm both in body and in mind before you continue.

CONTINUE: Proceed to deep relaxation from the large muscles to the tendons, to internal organs and finally to the bone marrow.

Other exercises such as the one described in the earlier chapter called Positive Imagery can also be done at this point.

You can now try to do the exercises explained so far or wait until after reading the entire book. Once you are comfortable with the exercises, you can then go on to the Dao Yin form. But first, you need to know about the...

Points and areas of the body

In this Dao Yin exercise routine, you'll be using the following vital points and areas.

Tiger's Mouth (Hu Kou)

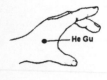

Fig. 10

Location

This refers to a wide *area* of the hand between the thumb and the index finger. It includes the Lung (Yin) and Colon (Yang) meridians. Together it allows the function of this paired Yin and Yang partner meridian to exert their synergistic functions.

Reasons why used

- Lung Meridian (Yin) governs Chi. It is in charge of respiration, the descending and dispersing of Chi and opens in the nose and throat.
- Colon meridian (Yang) receives food, transforms and transports food Chi. The Colon Chi also allows fluids to be absorbed and stools to be excreted.

Functions

Air and Food Chi are two of the three sources of Chi (Food, Air and inherited Chi) that combine to form the total Chi of the body. Therefore this partnership of Air and Food Chi is crucial to the overall makeup, quality, movement and existence of Chi in the body.

Self-massage with acupressure

The Tiger's Mouth includes Colon 4 (He Gu), a major point located on the back of the hand, just off the bone half way on the second metacarpal bone which is the part between the wrist and the knuckle that joins with the index finger. Use your thumb to apply pressure or massage to this point for any problems of the head and face such as headaches or acne. It is also good for the common cold, sore throat, fever, hay fever, toothache, tonsillitis and constipation. In the acupuncture point prescription formula, its calming action is successfully used to relieve stress, anxiety, tension or pain.

CAUTION: *Do not use on pregnant women because of its empirical function of promoting delivery during labour.*

Traditional acupuncture features

This is a Source (Yuan) point, and a major point used for all problems of the head and face. It is a special point for the invasion of Wind-Heat and relieves invasion of external symptoms such as Wind-Cold during the flu. It activates the dispersing function of the lung and stimulates intestinal function.

The Magpie Bridge (Que Chiao)

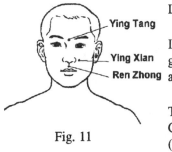

Fig. 11

Location

It is the *area* between the nostrils and the glabella, which is the part on the forehead just above the line of the eyebrows.

There are three major points in its proximity, Colon 20 (Ying Xian), Extra point Number 1 (Yin Tang) and Governor Vessel 26 (Ren Zhong).

Reasons why used

Used in Chi Kung, it is the place where the mind is focused prior to the start of breathing. This is said to facilitate the movement of Chi inside the body during inspiration.

Functions

- Colon 20 (Ying Xian) means welcome fragrance. It is located between the nasolabial grove and the midpoint of the lateral border of the nasal ala.
- Extra Point Number 1 called 'Seal Hall' (Yin Tang) is located on the midline of the body between the eyebrows. 'Seal' refers to the placing of a red mark between the eyebrows to represent wisdom and enlightenment and 'Hall' refers to the inner cranium which stores the mind.
- Governor Vessel 26 called 'centre of man' (Ren Zhong) is located on the mid-line of the body one-third the distance from the base of the nose to the top of the lip. The Governor Vessel meridian (master of Yang) travels up the spine, on top of the head and reaches this point which is on the Yin (front) part of the body. Ren Zhong refers to the area where the Yin and Yang on the body's midline (Conception and Governor Vessels) meet.

Self-Massage with acupressure

- Colon 20: A local point for nose problems, it is used for sinusitis, sneezing, runny or stuffy nose.
- Extra point Number 1: for frontal headaches, to increase concentration and reduce stress.
- Governor Vessel 26: A revival point used when unconscious.

Traditional acupuncture features

- Colon 20 facilitates the movement of Chi in and out of the lungs, clears the nose, dispels Wind, Wind-Cold and Wind-Heat and clears Heat that affect the olfactory function.
- Extra Point Number 1 is used to calm the mind, help focus and centre the mind. It harmonises the emotions and settles the Spirit.

- Governor Vessel 26 clears the mind, calms the spirit, restores collapsed Yang, regulates Governing Vessel and it is a major revival point.

Elixir or cinnabar field (Dan Tian)

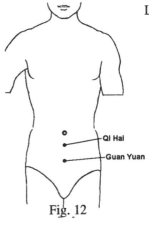

Fig. 12

Location

The Elixir Field is an *area* about the size of your palm (approximately three inches) when placed on the front midline of your body, on the Conception vessel, one inch below your umbilicus.

The Elixir Field includes the influence of two major points in the body, Conception Vessel 4 (Guan Yuan) and 6 (Qi Hai). Conception Vessel 4 (Guan Yuan) is located three inches below the umbilicus on the anterior mid-line of the body. Conception Vessel 6 (Qi Hai) is located one-and-a-half inches above Conception Vessel 4.

Reasons why used

- The elixir is a hypothetical life-prolonging substance for which Taoists have been searching for millennia.
- Ancient Taoist alchemists originally thought that the elixir was something physical which could be prepared from herbs or chemicals. They believed that the proper preparation and ingestion of the mineral cinnabar (hence the name cinnabar field) is able to impart immortality because of its near perfect balance of Yin and Yang and ability to nourish Source Chi. Source Chi is stored in the area between points Conception Vessel 4 and 7, the latter located at one inch below the umbilicus.
- This mineral also symbolised the state of open consciousness that is experienced during meditation.
- After thousands of years of study and experimentation, they found that the elixir is in fact inside the human body. In other words, if you want to prolong your life, you must find the elixir in your body, and then learn to nourish and

protect it.

Functions

- The Conception Vessel is the Master of Yin in the body. Its main functions are to distribute, control and regulate Yin Chi in the body. It balances the body at the centre (hence keeping us 'centred'), nourishes the sexual organs, controls and regulates growth and maturity.
- It is believed that the Dan Tian holds a major influence on the performance and health of the entire body and, eventually, your life.
- After respiration, the Chi inhaled is directed to Dan Tian. Chi is stored, mixed with the body's Source Chi and redistributed throughout the entire body.

Self-massage with acupressure

This is a special technique used to combine the effects of both points. Using your palm or fingers, massage up and down on a straight line from Conception Vessel 4 (Guan Yuan) to Conception Vessel 6 (Qi Hai) to help you with any type of menstrual or genital (male and female) problems, low energy or vitality, and to promote longevity.

CAUTION: *Avoid pressure on pregnant women.*

Traditional acupuncture features

- Conception Vessel 4 (Guan Yuan): Called the gate of origin, this point influences the amount of Source Chi that would pass through the Elixir Field. It adjusts the circulation of Chi and increases the Yang energy of the body. While being a major tonification point for the whole body, it can also restore collapsed Yin or Yang. Self-massage to tonify Chi and Blood (Yin) and to strengthen the body and mind.
- Conception Vessel 6 (Qi Hai): Called the Sea of Chi where the Source Chi gathers like a reservoir, it regulates the circulation of Chi and strengthens all the Yin organs. It is a major point for activating the production of blood or tonifying the whole body. Self-massage to increase Chi and Yang in the body during physical and mental exhaustion and depression.

Kidney 1 (Yong Quan)—bubbling or gushing spring

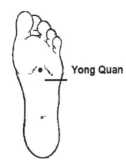

Yong Quan

Fig. 13

Location

On the soles of the feet in the centre of the crease when the toes are flexed.

Reasons why used

- This is the first *point* of the Kidney meridian. The description of the point according to traditional Chinese teaching suggests the source of fresh and active energy. From here the Chi of the Kidney meridian flows upward and outward like that of a bubbling or gushing spring.
- The main functions of the Kidney Chi are to store Essence (Yin) and govern birth, growth and reproduction (Yang). The kidney rules the reception of Chi from the Lungs. It also holds the balance between Fire and Water (Yin and Yang).
- Chinese medical theory holds that the Kidney Chi most usually and likely becomes deficient and depleted. Kidney Yin is the material foundation for Kidney Yang which is the exterior manifestation of Kidney Yin.
- As the Kidney Chi supports the Heart and because the Heart houses the Shen (Spirit), it calms the mind and the heart, especially when there is Fire in the head. Fire usually creates internal wind which can scatter the Spirit.

Functions

This is a major point to tonify the Yin in the body. It is the most Yin point on the body which is in constant contact with Earth, which is also Yin. Being on the sole of the foot it has a strong sinking action, therefore it is able to bring down the Fire or Heat in the head.

Self-massage with acupressure

Use your thumb to apply pressure on this point for heat stroke, insomnia, high fever, hypertension, fainting (with the person lying down), convulsions and shock to promote resuscitation.

Traditional acupuncture features

This point opens the sensory orifices and calms the spirit. It tonifies Yin, clears Heat, subdues Wind, calms the mind and restores consciousness.

Pericardium 8 (Lao Gong)

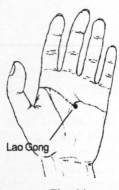

Lao Gong

Fig. 14

Location

On the Pericardium channel, in the centre of the palm, when the fist is clenched, the *point* lies between the tips of the middle and ring fingers.

Reasons why used

In Chinese medicine, the Spirit resides in the Heart. The Pericardium acts as a protector to the Heart, there-fore protecting the Spirit as well. Called the 'Palace of Labour', this point is involved in physical, mental and Spiritual revitalisation.

Functions

It is the most effective point to cool and clear Heart Fire. Many Pericardium points have a powerful influence on the mental and emotional state.

Self-massage with acupressure

To revive consciousness, promote heart function and circulation of blood, for

108

tongue ulcers and brain function disorders such as epilepsy.

Traditional acupuncture features

It cools Heat in the blood, removes Wind in the Heart due to the rising of Fire and calms the Spirit. Regulates Heart Chi, especially of excess Chi and Yang, revives consciousness and clears the brain.

Governor Vessel 4 (Ming Men)

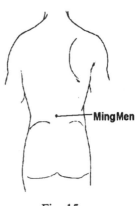

Fig. 15

Location

Governor Vessel 4 point is located on the spine, between the spinous process of the second and third lumbar vertebra. It exerts an influence to an area that covers seven centimetres below the point to correspond to the Elixir Field on the front of the body.

Reasons why used

This point means the 'Yang or Vital Gate'. In Taoism, this is the area on the Governor Vessel meridian which runs along the spine on the back of the body (Yang), that corresponds to the Elixir Field which is situated on the front of the body (Yin). It nourishes and stabilises the functions of the Kidneys and the Elixir Field. That area involves this point.

Functions

The Governor Vessel is the master of Yang in the body. Its main functions are to provide a place for all the Yang meridians of the body to meet, to regulate and consolidate the functions of these Yang meridians. Likewise the Yang meridians affect the Governor Vessel. It influences the adrenal glands and the sympathetic nervous system and affects mental energy.

This area is considered a passageway for Source Chi, Kidney Chi and Essence which depending on their relative strength or weakness, make up the body's fundamental vitality level.

Self-massage with acupressure

It is the most powerful point to increase overall Yang in the body; therefore can be used for overall weakness or feeling of cold. It is also good for Kidney problems such as nephritis, sexual dysfunctions such as impotence or sterility, and back pain.

CAUTION: *Avoid pressure on pregnant women.*

Traditional acupuncture features

In Chinese medicine, the Governor Vessel meridian is regarded as the regulator of Chi and Yang in the body. Therefore this area tonifies and increases Kidney Chi, especially its Yang aspect. It also tonifies the Yang Chi of the whole body. It strengthens the back, is a major tonification point of the whole body and is effectively used in overall weakness.

Governor Vessel 20 (Bai Hui)

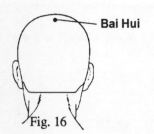

Bai Hui

Fig. 16

Location

This *point* is located on the midline of the head where a line connecting the tips of both ears crosses the vertex of the head.

Reasons why used

This is the uppermost point, the Yang pole of the

body. It is a major point in the circle of energy.

Functions

Called 'One hundred meetings', it is a point where all the Yang channels in the body meet. Therefore it regulates the Yang Chi in the body and it is quite powerful in raising Yang and lifting the Spirit, especially when depressed.

Self-massage with acupressure

Lifts the Spirit, raises energy when depleted, fainting, headache, vertigo, forgetfulness, shock, seizures and promotes resuscitation.

CAUTION: *Avoid pressure on children.*

Traditional acupuncture features

Prolapse of any kind such as that of the uterus or rectum, spreads Liver Chi, subdues Liver Yang, and extinguishes Liver Wind. Restores collapsed Yang.

Let us now look at the stances that are used in the Dao Yin form...

Stances

Stance training helps to promote good blood circulation. It strengthens the muscles in your legs. It teaches you balance, correct posture and allows the blood to quickly return back to your heart for re-oxygenation.

All stances are performed with the following rules:

- spine is straight
- shoulders are fully relaxed
- elbows are slightly bent to allow the arm to form a circle
- except where indicated, the knees are always bent
- muscles of the whole palm are relaxed; yet the palm is sensitive and able to feel or project energy
- Tiger's mouth and the rest of the palm expresses the formation of a circle
- mind is fully calm
- let your subconscious mind take over
- your hips are the key to your movements.

The following stances are used in the Dao Yin form. Please study them carefully as they are the foundation to the form.

Ready stance

Feet together, knees slightly bent, spine straight, arms at the side of the body, shoulders relaxed, elbows slightly bent, palms relaxed but sensitive and facing the side of your thighs.

- Relax body, calm mind.
- Thought is concentrated on Dan Tian point.
- Feel at ease and ready to do the exercises.

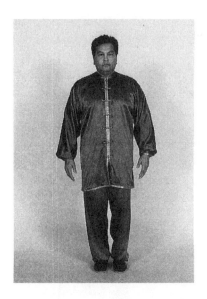

Fig. 17

Opening stance

- Toes face front.
- Palms by the side.
- Finger tips facing down.
- Body erect and relaxed.
- Feet are parallel with each other.
- Distance between the feet is the same width as your shoulders.
- Weight of the whole body is sunk to the floor.
- Body and mind are in a completely relaxed state and operate as one.

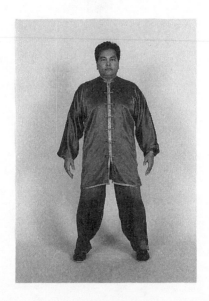

Fig. 18

Horse stance

The distance between both feet is approximately three-and-a-half times the length of your foot. Similar measurement can be achieved at one-and-a-half times the width of your shoulders.

- Both knees are bent.
- Spine is erect.

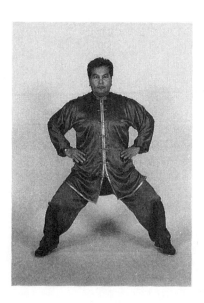

Fig. 19

Bow stance

- 70 percent of the weight of your body is on the front leg.
- Back leg is straight and bears the remainder 30 percent of the body weight.
- Chest faces squarely forward.
- Distance between the feet is no less than that of a horse stance with one leg placed forward.

When forming bow stance, do not raise buttocks. Relax hips and drop buttocks. Keep the back heel on the ground.

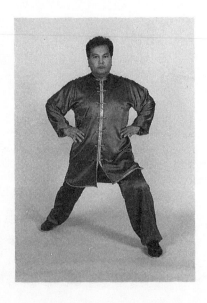

Fig. 20

Heel stance

Ninety percent of your body weight is held on the back leg. The front leg is straight, the knee is not bent, toes point upwards. The chest faces forward.

When forming Heel stance, keep your trunk straight. Relax waist and do not raise but shrink your buttocks. This is easily done by thrusting your hips forward.

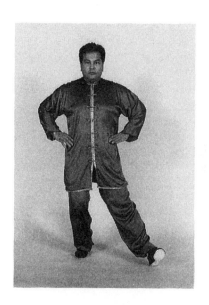

Fig. 21

Cross step kneeling stance

Front leg:
- Toes are squarely facing front.
- Holds 50 percent of your body weight.
- Knees are bent.

Back leg:
- Crosses at the back of the front leg.
- Holds the remaining 50 percent of the body weight.
- This leg is supported by the ball of the foot.
- Do not allow the heel of this leg to touch the floor.
- Both legs tightly intertwined together.

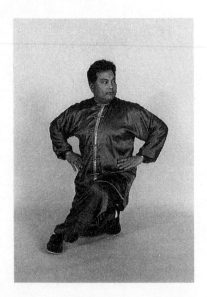

Fig. 22

Holding the Moon

- Breathing exercise with meditation.
- Focus on Lao Gong point and Dan Tian.

This exercise is best done with your eyes closed. Breathe deeply and slowly from your Dan Tian point.

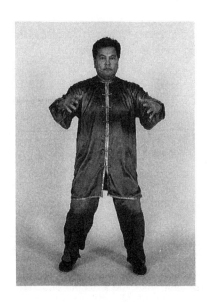

Fig. 23

The Dao Yin form— health protection skill

Now that you understand the stances used, here's the Dao Yin set of exercises to help you to be in a state of harmony, balance and calmness.

These exercises are called Dao Yin Yang Sheng Gong Bao Jian Gong and follow the principles of modern Dao Yin as taught by my teacher Professor Zhang Guang-de of the People's Republic of China.

Theory is the Yin side of knowledge, practice is the Yang, so it is important for you to study both the theory and practice of the techniques because each one helps the other and one cannot do without the other.

So far, you have learnt the theoretical and mental skills; now it is time for the physical skills so that you can balance Yin and Yang and move Chi.

This is an introduction to Dao Yin exercises. The explanations will assist you to gain the benefits of Dao Yin.

If you would like to gain the full benefits, then you must seek professional instruction from a competent and experienced master or teacher.

A master-teacher will ensure that your movements are correct and that the transition from one technique to another is correct. The internal feelings of the exercises and his or her personal experience of the exercises will help to perfect your techniques and give you a deeper understanding of the art.

These techniques contain an enormous amount of power which can only be fully developed by an experienced practitioner.

120

Please study the whole instruction before doing the form.

Some tips to consider when doing the exercises

The keys to receiving the benefits of Dao Yin exercises are:

- Ensure points Lung 9 (Fig. 8) and Heart 7 (Fig. 9) are felt in all movements.
- Your mind must focus on the vital points or areas designated especially for each exercise before your body starts to move.
- Breathe correctly during all movements.
- Always start the exercises with the left side.
- Use your inner power instead of the strength of your outer physical muscles. This uses the theory of 'Inner Intent—Outer Stillness'.
- Your torso leads all movements. Do not move your arms independently of the rest of your body. Your arms move around and with your 'centre' as the earth orbits around the sun. Your whole body always moves as one unit.
- All parts of your body rotate in circles or arcs.
- Your mind can focus slightly ahead of the current movement to help the body learn to follow the energy of the mind.
- Your arms and legs move at the same time.
- Avoid shallow breathing and breathe smoothly to your Dan Tian point (just below the navel).

It has recently come to light in western medicine that the joints are not to be locked when performing exercises. Chinese study of physiology long ago realised that locking a joint leads to multiple trauma of that joint. This can lead to arthritis and other conditions which may cause pain, deformity or permanent reduction in mobility. So keep all your joints slightly bent during exercises.

Weight transfer

The transfer of weight from one leg to another is critically important. At all times you should endeavour to create a continuous circle while transferring weight. For example, when the weight is on both legs, transfer all the body weight on to one leg, then slowly move the other leg weightlessly along the ground, then shift the weight gradually and slowly by attempting to create a smooth flow and transfer of energy from one leg to another.

Directions

Throughout the form please follow the directions and angles as described below.

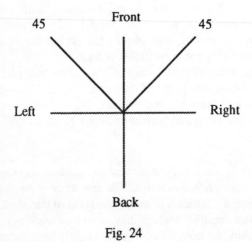

Fig. 24

Mental preparation before commencing the form

Your body

- Place your tongue against the roof of your mouth.
- Close your mouth, lips together but not tense.
- Straighten your body, lift the chest.
- Relax your shoulders and arms.
- Your neck and head erect.

- Relax and feel every muscle fibre from your head to your toe.
- Feel comfortable with the weight of your whole body resting on your feet.
- Breate in and out through your nose.

Your mind

- Close your eyes and calm your mind.
- Regulate your breathing with your mind focusing on Dan Tian.
- Recite the exercise formula:

> *' Throw away your troubles in the stillness of the night.
> Thought on Dan Tian and seal the orifices. Breathe gently and
> connect the magpie bridge. Light as a swallow flying in the
> sky'.*

Then allow your sub-conscious mind to take over your conscious mind.
After eight abdominal breaths, open your eyes and feel ready to exercise.

Skill No. 1: Adjust breathing

Vital points used: Yong Quan (fig. 13) and Lao Gong (fig. 14).
- Adopt a Ready Stance.
- Inhale and step your left foot to the left to form an opening stance.
- Exhale and let your weight sink to the ground.

Step A
- Inhaling deeply and smoothly to your Dan Tian point, contracting and raising Hui Yin.
- Raise your arms forward and upward to shoulder level with your arms the same width as your shoulders and palms facing the floor (fig. 25).
- While raising your arms, lean forward and press on Yong Chuan point located in the ball of your foot. Keep your heels on the ground at all times (fig. 26).

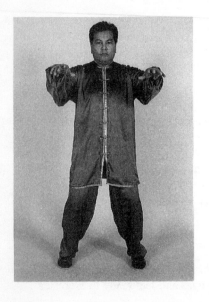

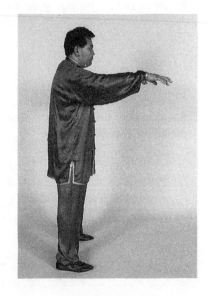

Fig. 25   Fig. 26

Step B
* Exhaling, relaxing your belly and Hui Yin.
* Bend your legs and lower your arms to the level of your Dan Tian (figs. 27 & 28). Figure 28 is a side view.
* This is done by drawing back and dropping your elbows, your fingertips slightly facing up and your palms pressing down. Then continue raising your arms as in Step A.

Steps A and B constitute one whole exercise, totalling two counts.

Key Points:
* Drop your elbows and shoulders.
* Do not thrust your belly out.
* When bending, relax your waist.
* Concentrate your thought on Dan Tian.
* Do the whole exercise 16 times.

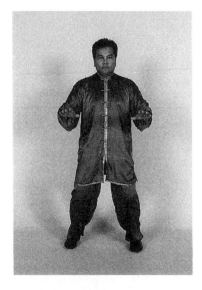

Fig. 27

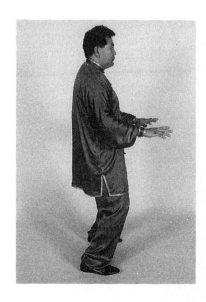

Fig. 28

Skill No. 2: Push the boat downstream

Vital point used: Lao Gong (fig. 14).

Step A
- Inhaling deeply and smoothly to your Dan Tian point, contracting and raising your Hui Yin.
- On an opening stance, turn your body at the waist to face left 45 degrees, do not move your knees or feet (fig. 29).
- Bend your knees and shift your weight onto your right leg.
- Raise both your arms to the level of your shoulders (just like in Skill No. 1) while stepping your left foot forward left 45 into a heel stance (fig. 30). Then pull back both your arms to arrive near the chest.

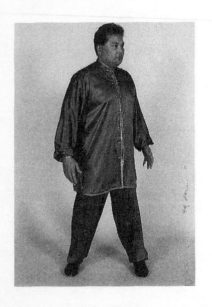

Fig. 29

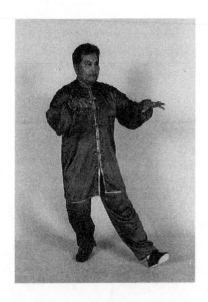

Fig. 30

Step B
- Exhaling, relaxing your belly and Hui Yin.
- Put your left foot firmly on the ground, transfer your weight onto your left leg to form a left bow stance while pushing your palms downward, forward and slightly upward to end at the same level as your shoulders. The distance between both your arms is the same width as your shoulders.
- Move as if pushing a boat downstream, giving yourself a feeling of ease and grace. Look ahead left 45 degrees (fig. 31).

Step C: Transition step
- Stay in the same spot, bend the right knee and transfer weight back to form a heel stance while pulling both your arms back to the chest to recommence step B.
- To finish off, with arms moving to the front of your body, palms facing down, turn slightly rightward to look at the right hand and face front starting position (fig. 32).
- Draw left foot in to meet the right and return both your arms to the ready stance position.

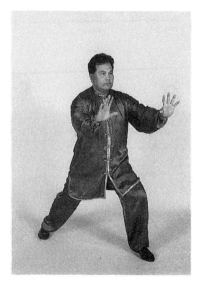

Fig. 31

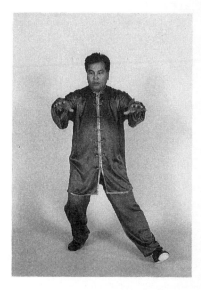

Fig. 32

Key Points

- Steps A and B constitute the whole exercise. For left side, do three times plus one transition step. Repeat the same for the right side.
- When pushing your palms forward, drop shoulders, relax elbows, lower wrists and tilt up finger tips. Coordinate with the movement of your legs. This is expressed with the tradition of ' Beginning at the root, smooth in the middle and reaching the tip'.
- Your thought is concentrated on your Lao Gong point (middle of palm).

Skill No. 3: Carry the sun and moon on the shoulder

Vital point used: Ming Men (fig. 15).

Step A

- Inhaling deep and smoothly to your Dan Tian point, contracting and raising Hui Yin.
- Start with a ready stance, turn your torso 90 degrees left to face back. Raising both your arms upwards to shoulder level, rotate your arms inward as far as possible to have your thumbs pointing downwards. Continue turning your palm to face upwards. Look at your left hand (fig. 33). Figure 33 is a side view.

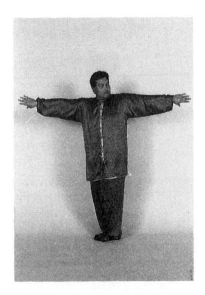

Fig. 33

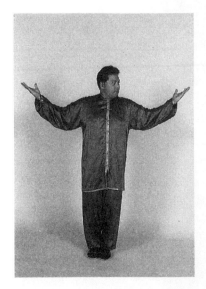

Fig. 34

- When your palms reach shoulder level, turn both palms to face upwards (your right palm is rotated in a clockwise motion and your left palm in an anti-clockwise motion to face upwards). Bend your elbows. Keep the angle between your upper arm and torso to just under 90 degrees and the angle between the upper arm and forearm to about 100 degrees (fig. 34).
- Keep your palms still, facing upwards and your finger tips sidewards. Keep looking at the left palm.

Step B

- Exhaling, relaxing your belly and Hui Yin.
- Begin returning torso to starting position while looking at the left palm until you face the front, then look forward. Your left arm should be pointing towards the left and your right arm towards the right (fig. 35).
- Turn your palms to face front, fingertips upwards and bring your arms to the front in line with your shoulders.
- Drag your arms in an arc downwards to end in a ready stance position (fig. 36).

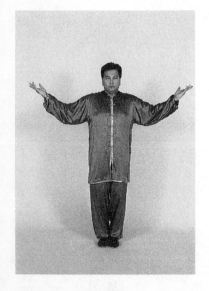

Fig. 35

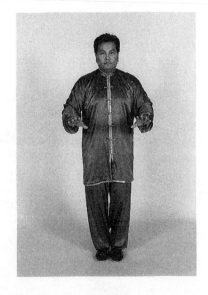

Fig. 36

Key points

- Steps A and B constitute two counts. Do this exercise alternatively left and then right side to a total of 16 times.
- When forming as if carrying the sun and moon on the shoulder, relax your waist and stretch your body. Drop your shoulders and lower your elbows. Your hands are above your shoulders, elbows below your shoulders.
- Visualise one arm as if holding the sun, the other as if holding the moon. The radiance of the sun and the moon warms the vital organs and nourishes the heart.
- The aim is to eventually turn the waist fully to 90 degrees. At first you may not be able to turn fully, so persevere. It is important that you do not turn past the point of pain. Keep your torso erect. Do not lose your balance.
- Thought is concentrated on your Ming Men point (on the spine near the lower back).

Skill No. 4: A Roc spreads its wings

Vital point used: Dan Tian (fig. 12).

Place both palms on the front of your Dan Tian with palms facing upward and finger tips facing each other. The distances between the finger tips of both your hands and between your palms and body are all about 10 centimetres. This is roughly the width of the widest part of the hand from the thumb to the little finger. Look straight ahead (fig. 37).

Step A

- Inhaling deeply and smoothly to your Dan Tian point, contracting and raising Hui Yin.

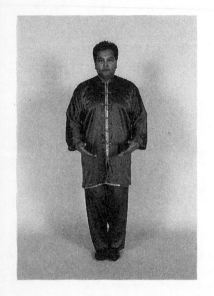

Fig. 37

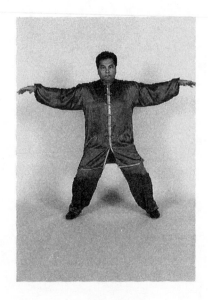

Fig. 38

- Shift your weight onto your right leg, squat your right leg and step your left foot to the left into a horse stance. At the same time, stretch out your arms to the side (left and right). As you straighten both your legs, share weight equally between both your legs (fig. 38). Continue moving both your arms upward in an arc to above your head, palms facing upward and finger tips facing each other as if spreading the wings slowly (fig. 39).
- Look straight ahead.

Step B (return back to fig. 37)

- Exhaling, relaxing your belly and Hui Yin.
- Squat both your legs into a horse stance while lowering both arms to shoulder level, pointing towards left and right (fig. 38).
- Shift your weight onto your right leg, return the left foot to meet the right foot, then straighten both legs. At the same time, drop both palms in an arc to return to the front of your Dan Tian. Both palms face upwards and your body weight is now on both legs (fig. 37).

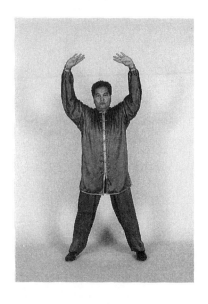

Fig. 39

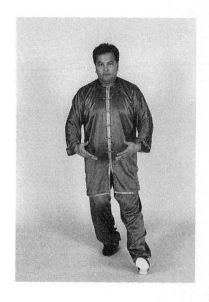

Fig. 40

- Repeat steps A and B on the right side.

Step C

- Inhaling, contracting and raising your Hui Yin.
- Shift your weight onto your right foot, bend your right leg and step your left foot to the front to form a heel stance (fig. 40).
- Transfer your weight slowly onto your left foot into a bow stance while raising both arms in an arc forward to shoulder level. Your palms now face your body (fig. 41).
- Straighten both legs and lift up your right heel off the ground
- Raise both arms upwards while turning the palms anti-clockwise to face up above your head. Look straight ahead (fig. 42).
- The ball of your right foot is used for support and balance.

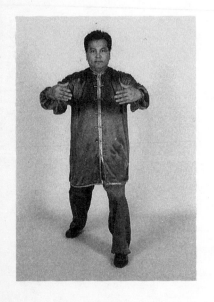 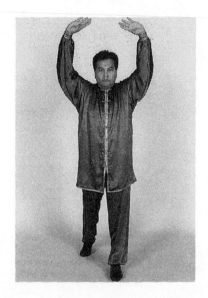

Fig. 41   Fig. 42

134

Step D (return back to fig. 37)

- Exhaling, relaxing your belly and Hui Yin.
- In this part reverse Step C.
- Shift your weight onto your right leg and let your right heel return to the ground. Lower your palms to face your head, then shift your weight onto the heel stance. Finally your left foot returns to meet your right foot with both palms returned to the starting position, both palms face upwards and look straight ahead.

Repeat Steps C and D with your right leg.

Key Points:

- Concentrate your thought on the Dan Tian point.
- When holding up your palms above your head, relax your waist and stretch your body. Lift up the heel of your back foot as much as possible, press the ball of that foot on the ground to massage your Yong Quan point. When holding palms in front of your Dan Tian draw in the chest slightly and breathe out.
- Try to move your legs and arms at the same time.
- Steps A, B, C and D should be done twice.

Skill No. 5: Lift up a millstone

Vital point used: Dan Tian (fig. 12).

Step A

- Inhaling deeply and smoothly to your Dan Tian point, contracting and raising Hui Yin.
- From the position at the commencement of Skill 4, look at both palms while raising them up to the level of your shoulder. Keep them facing upwards. Turn both your palms naturally to face the front, gently extend both your arms to the side while you shift all your weight onto your right leg and step your left foot into a horse stance to the left (fig. 43).

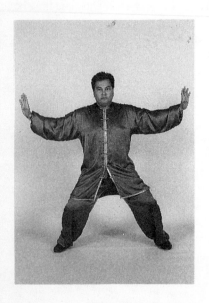

Fig. 43

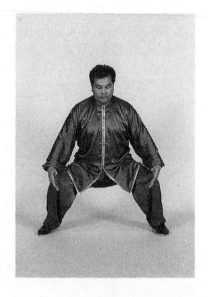

Fig. 44

Step B

- Exhaling, relaxing your belly and Hui Yin.
- Arms from shoulder level, turn palms to face down, move your arms downward in a curve (along the left-right line) to arrive just in front of the knees while the legs bend to a horse stance (fig. 44).
- Your arms form a circle with palms facing upward and finger tips facing each other. Imagine holding up a large stone. Do not curl your spine or lower your head.

Step C

- Inhaling deeply and smoothly to your Dan Tian point, contracting and raising Hui Yin.
- Use your legs and waist to push your body up while you raise both your palms up as if lifting a large millstone. Your palms arrive at the front of the chest. Palms still face upwards and finger tips facing each other. Look straight ahead (fig. 45).
- Continue to extend both your arms to the side at shoulder level as in Step A.

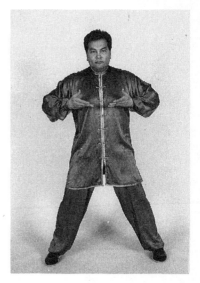

Fig. 45

Transition Step:

- From Step C transfer your weight on your right leg and bring your left leg to meet the right.

Key Points:

- Concentrate your thought on the Dan Tian point.
- When bending down, do not lower your head or bend the body. Keep your back straight.
- When standing up, use your head to raise the body by raising your head to the sky, drop your shoulders.

137

- When moving your palms upward as if holding a millstone, the requirement is: 'Holding not with force but with thought.'
- Do steps A, B and C three times plus one transition step. Repeat the same for the right side.

Skill No. 6: Push the window open to look at the moon

Vital point used: Lao Gong (fig. 14).

Step A

- Inhaling deeply and smoothly to your Dan Tian point, contracting and raising Hui Yin.
- Form a ready stance and turn your waist to face left.
- Move your right arm across the front of your body and raise it to left shoulder while the left arm is raised to the left to stop at shoulder level.
- Look at the left palm.
- Both hands have thumbs facing down, that is, the left palm faces back and the right palm faces front (fig. 46).

Step B

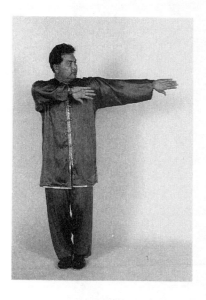

Fig. 46

- Exhaling, relaxing belly and Hui Yin.
- Bend the knees and lower the body, turn your torso to the right while swinging both palms forward in an arc, in front of you, to the right. This time the right palm faces the front and the left palm faces the back. The left arm is near the right elbow while the right arm is extended. Look at your right palm (figs. 47 & 48).
- Shift your weight to your right foot and half bend your right leg.
- Step your left foot to the left forming a Bow stance (fig. 49).

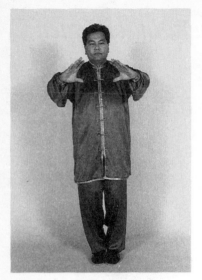

Fig. 47

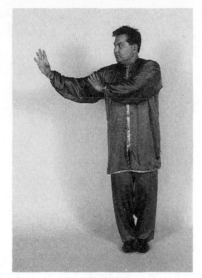

Fig. 48

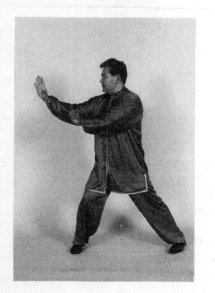

Fig. 49

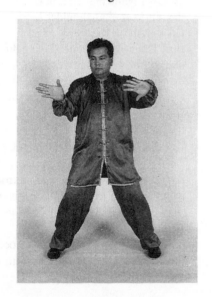

Fig. 50

Step C

- Inhaling deeply and smoothly to your Dan Tian point, contracting and raising Hui Yin.
- Use the ball of your left foot as an axis to turn your left heel making your left toes face the front. Then shift your weight to the left foot.
- Drag both palms from the right to the front of the body. The palms face the front. The angles of the palms are such that all fingertips face right (fig. 50).
- Start to cross your right foot to the back of your left foot into a cross leg kneeling stance.
- Look at the right palm and continue to move both palms to the left.

Step D

- Exhaling, relaxing your belly and Hui Yin.
- Squat down as low as you can on both legs to form a cross-leg kneeling stance. Your right heel if off the floor. Continue to push both palms to the left, finger tips of both hands to face the front. Continue turning your waist to the left.
- The left arm raises to above the head and the right arm pushes along the left line level to your navel as if pushing open the window to look at the moon. Look straight left between both hands (fig. 51).

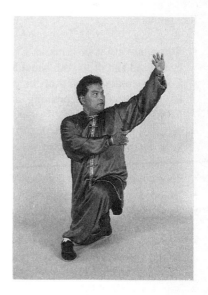

Fig. 51

Transition to right side

- Inhale deeply and smoothly to your Dan Tian point, contract and raise anus.
- Do not move from the cross-leg stance.
- Circle both arms down to just in front of your knees (fig. 52),
- Slowly stand up and raise both your arms like in step A, the right leg moves from the cross-leg stance to meet your left toe to form a ready stance.

Key points

- When moving your arms in a curve, be relaxed and drop your shoulders.
- Coordinate the forming of the cross-leg stance with the pushing of the palm.
- When forming the cross-leg stance, keep torso erect and keep both legs tightly together.

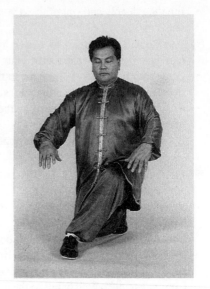

Fig. 52

- Thought is concentrated on Lao Gong point.
- Do not attempt to go too low in the cross-leg stance at first.
- Turn body smoothly to the side throughout descent into the Cross-Leg Kneeling Stance.
- Do Steps A, B, C, and D on the left side, then do the transition step to repeat A, B, C and D on the right side.
- Do the A, B, C and D steps twice on the left side and twice on the right side.

Skill No. 7: Brush the dust in the wind

Vital point used: Lao Gong (fig. 14).

Step A

- Inhaling deeply and smoothly to your Dan Tian point while contracting and raising Hui Yin.
- Turn your torso left 45 degrees. Rotate and raise both arms up to your side to reach shoulder level so that thumbs face down. Bring both of your arms to front, naturally straightened (fig. 53).
- Turn your right palm clockwise and left palm anti-clockwise.
- Raise all fingers to face the sky, keep rotating your wrist in a circle while you bring the back of the last three fingers of both hands to your chest.
- At the same time shift your weight onto the right foot, bend your right leg, turn body left 45 and step left foot left 45 to form a left Heel stance.

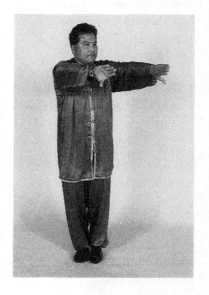

Fig. 53

- With both arms near the body, slightly brush the body (the dust) downwards along the rib cage (fig. 54).

Step B

- Exhaling, relaxing your belly and Hui Yin.
- As you transfer weight forward onto the left leg into Bow Stance, rotate both palms outward, swing both arms out wide to the side, then upwards to the front to reach the level of the shoulder. The thumbs are now facing down.

143

Look straight ahead on the bow stance left 45 degrees (fig. 55).

Transition

- Bring the back of the last three fingers of your hands to lightly touch the chest while you lean back onto your right leg to form a heel stance. Spread both your arms to your sides and return your arms to the front of your body while your left leg returns to meet your right leg.

Key Points

- Your thought is concentrated on Lao Gong.
- Do steps A and B three times plus one transition. Repeat on the right side.

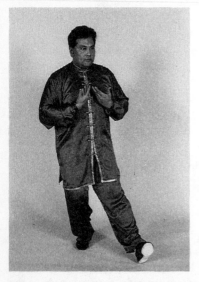

Fig. 54

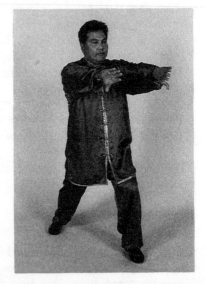

Fig. 55

Skill No. 8: Old man strokes beard

Vital points used: Dan Tian (fig. 12) and
Bai Hui (fig. 16).

Step A

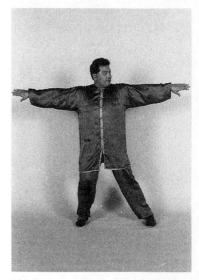

- Inhaling deeply and smoothly to your
Dan Tian point, contracting and raising
Hui Yin.
- Adopt the ready stance. Shift weight
onto the right leg and bend it. Step out
left foot to the left side at a distance
twice the width of your opening stance.
Look at your left palm at the same time
rotate and raise both arms to the sides
with palms facing back and thumbs
down at shoulder level (fig. 56).

Step B

Fig. 56

- Exhaling, relaxing belly and anus.
- Move your right leg to join up with your left leg. Rotate arms to make palms
face the front, thumbs face up and bend the elbows slightly (fig. 57). Bend
your wrists to bring your arms close to the face, all fingertips pointing at the
chin and palms facing the body (fig. 58). With your Tiger's mouth holding
the imaginary beard, push both palms downward in a circular motion away
from the body as though stroking the beard until palms reach the level of
Dan Tian while gradually straightening legs (fig. 59).

145

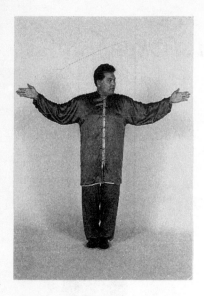

Fig. 57

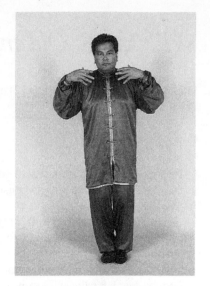

Fig. 58

Key Points

- Repeat steps A and B with the right leg.
- Do steps A and B twice.
- Look to the side to which you are stepping.
- Then repeat the whole movement by standing still, on the same spot, with the left and right legs. In other words stay on the ready stance, in the same spot and do the arm movements of A and B twice. Look to the front during the whole of this section. Breathe out very slowly as you slowly 'stroke beard'.
- Your thought is concentrated on Dan Tian point.

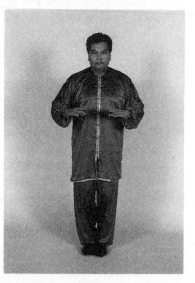

Fig. 59

- When pressing down both palms, lift up Bai Hui point (crown of the head), giving the impression of radiating vigour.
- When finishing the whole series of eight exercises, do eight full breathing cycles and remain calm for a little while before leaving the exercise position.

Finishing the Form.

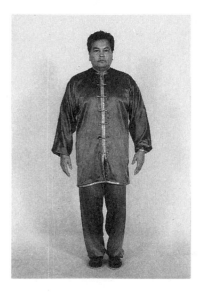

Return both your arms to your side to form a ready stance (fig. 60). Then close your eyes and do eight full deep Dan Tian breaths. After that, open your eyes and make sure that you remain calm for a few minutes after the exercise.

Fig. 60

Part IV: YOUR JOURNEY FORWARD

Lessons about living

'Follow the ancient way,
To master the present.
Knowing the ancient way
Is the key to the Tao.'

Tao Te Ching, Chapter 14

Now that you are capable of regaining and maintaining your physical, mental, emotional and spiritual health, you will be able to direct your life with more purpose. Taoism provides a general philosophy to guide your conscience. This philosophy is based on what is right and wrong in the natural world rather than what is legal or illegal in our society. When using your energies, apply the life-loving philosophy of Taoism for both personal and universal advancement.

Caring for the Universe begins with caring for ourselves

The way in which people care for their bodies often reflects their attitudes towards the environment; and vice versa is also true. If we do not respect and keep our body healthy, we will not do the same for the Universe around us.

The western approach to health bears a strong resemblance to the 'avalanche effect' discovered several years ago by scientists studying the causes of avalanches in Europe.

When it was realised that avalanches were occurring more and more frequently in 200 to 400 year old villages, which had historically been free of avalanches, an international body of scientists was assigned the task of finding

150

the causes. Investigations found that there were no longer enough trees on the mountains to stop heavy snow from sliding downhill. The trees which had previously prevented this from happening had been killed off by acid rain. The acid rain was a direct result of chemical pollution pumped into the atmosphere in Europe's heavy industrial areas located many hundreds of miles away.

When you trace the chain of causation back to the beginning, it is easy to see the links. However, without the benefit of hindsight, when looking at industrial pollution and smoke going into the atmosphere you would not predict an increase in the number of avalanches in a distant country the following year.

Similarly when you start smoking you do not pick up a cigarette and think: 'This will give me lung cancer'. But later on, when you have lung cancer, it is fairly easy to trace the chain of causation back to that first cigarette.

In neither case could you look at the end result and identify the beginning without scientific knowledge. But we do not have to know the end result, or have vast amounts of specialised knowledge, to know from the outset that our actions are wrong. When we pump pollution into the atmosphere we may not know the specific effect it is going to have, but deep down inside we know that it cannot be good. Our basic instincts tells us that pumping toxins and rubbish into the atmosphere, upon which all things rely for life, cannot be beneficial.

Taoists consider health to be physical, mental, emotional and spiritual fitness working in harmony within the individual. Mind and body are not separated: they both exist and work in unison. This synergy allows the individual to maximise performance in each of those aspects. Consequently, the individual develops a greater ability to maintain health and prevent disease.

By adopting a similar attitude you will find it far easier to identify and avoid harmful substances, personal habits, people and situations. Eventually your need for western medical treatment with drugs, which is largely concerned with the treatment of established physical illness, will be greatly reduced.

Is it right or is it wrong?

You do not need to go into the chemistry or geology and all the rest of it to apply the simple question 'Is this right or wrong?'. Any person who can make a decision between right or wrong would know whether they should continue to do these things to themselves and their environment.

It is the same with whaling, drift netting, logging of the rainforests, cruelty to animals and all the other crimes we commit against the environment and other people. It is a simple question of whether our actions are right or wrong, not can we justify it? Does our economy rely on it? Are we going to destroy industry and jobs? Those questions are simply distractions from the real issue: is it right or is it wrong?

If our actions are wrong we may be fortunate enough not to have to pay for our stupidity and greed. But our children and grandchildren will pay the price with compound interest, and we will have wasted irreplaceable treasures.

Greed is a negative emotion (Yin). It is reflected in the body as Yin illness. There are many examples of monetary or cultural greed today. One example is seen in countries which continue to allow drift netting in the oceans. Their attitude to whaling is even more sad. Rich economies in the world with all the money at their disposal should take urgent measures to stop this cruel abuse of nature's gifts. The extensive cutting down of our rainforests is another. And so is hunger caused by poverty.

Taoism helps us appraise our place in nature and in the world, especially in the light of our current environmental and social crises and cruelty to animals. Again, it is just a matter of looking at the core issues. We know that we are heading in the wrong direction. We know that it cannot be right to offer the future of our descendants as collateral on a debt that we have no intention of repaying. The lesson here is simply: only do it if it is right. A balance needs to be struck.

Everything in our Universe has a right to life

We are a minutely small part of the Universe. To live on planet Earth means we must share our spaceship with all other inhabitants.

Modern humans do not consider themselves to be a part of the natural world. Instead, we sit on top of it and rule it. We do not live in it. The more civilised we become the more we tear ourselves away from the natural world. In some parts of the world, city dwellers take their children to the zoo to see a cow. I wonder how we can possibly live in our world harmoniously when we do not know what our world is.

As much as we like to tell ourselves that we do everything because of our intelligence and intellectual motivation, we still have basic animal instincts. We eat, breed, maintain personal security just as animals do. We are still mammals. We are still part of the animal kingdom.

In the animal kingdom each creature has a specific job to perform within their natural environment. Carnivores assist in maintaining the health and controlling the population of their prey. Small insects are responsible for the cross-pollination of plants. Birds carry seeds and protect plants from harmful insects. Every creature performs an essential task that suits its physical and mental ability.

The main difference between humans and other animals is that we have inherited the gift of a much greater mental capacity. Due to our higher intelligence we have the honour and privilege of maintaining harmony between the whole planet and everything on it. Our generation has totally neglected that responsibility. We have accepted many of the benefits of our intelligence but we have not used it for its true purpose.

An ant nest with its thousands of individual ants, is considered as one animal. Each and every ant works for the good of the nest. The bee hive is the same. So too is our society made up of millions of individuals and yet, from a

153

scientific point of view, like the ants and bees, we are one individual.

However, in our society the individual members work for their own self interest, usually at the expense of others. As a result of this the larger animal to which we all belong, society, is out of control and has lost its directions. It reminds me of a dog chasing its tail.

Summon your inner strength and use it

The chinese believe that hope, joy and purpose help you heal your body. Summon and use your inner strength, persevere and be determined to see yourself through the Yin (rough) patches of life. Take responsibility, do not use blame or self-pity and patiently wait for the Yang to come. It will, if you let it.

To grow mentally, emotionally and spiritually, to discover the true meaning of satisfaction, pleasure and happiness, help others in their quest. You have the strength to do that.

Peacefully accept your situation and work hard to improve it

In life, an example of Yin is the undesirable while Yang is the desirable. Rich or poor, *accept your path* in life without boasting or complaining. Boasting can turn a Yang situation into a Yin, for the ancients say that what is given can easily be taken away. Nature does not boast about the beauty it has given us. Complaining, on the other hand, does not turn the situation around. In fact it makes it worse with Yin becoming double Yin. To help you recognise the Tao in your life, accept with an open heart what is inevitable. Then you will be able to see the changes that take place.

154

Control your thoughts and emotions by accepting everything that comes along, without worry or excess joy. Learn to accept the inevitable because, whatever the future holds, no one can fight the universal laws or stop the fulfilment of Tao.

Believe in yourself that you can do it.

Respect, love and support others

Our ability to love and care for others depends on our connection with every part of our inner being, who we really are. This book helps you find your true nature to love and support others, without judgement and allow others to love and support you.

Let others follow their path at their speed. What is suitable for you is not always suitable for others.

Instead of comparing people or judging them against social expectations, affirm, enjoy and value people. See people as their own individual, separate from us and others. Believe in people and give them a go. People are more important than things. Put love and care in everything you touch, do or say.

Do good. Never harm others by thought or deed, irrespective of what they do or say. Words are the most powerful tools used by humans. So choose your words carefully.

Be willing to win and allow others to win too.

Time can change you...but you can't change time

Life is a sacred gift. It is your duty to care for and maintain your body so that it can help you enjoy this gift.

Greater health, physically, mentally and spiritually, provides you with more options because it increases your vision and capacity in any one or all of these three fields.

Having studied this book, you can now be responsible for the consequences of your actions. You now have greater skills and you no doubt realise your responsibility to your health and to the whole universe. You will see that with just a bit of effort from each of us and with the application of our technology and intelligence, we can easily fix today's problems. For example, we can immediately start by drastically cutting our defence budget and spend it on health, education, and programs that protect the environment.

It is *choice*, not chance, that will determine the outcome of your future and your planet. The results will be decided from the actions *you* take. Like the philosophy which found me, it is no accident you have come across the ancient healing secrets offered in this book. Use it. Use the wisdom of the Tao and your experiences to shape your present. Use the present to mould your future.

The Chinese say *'A journey of a thousand miles begins with one step'*. Now is the right time to start. Go forth, and may the power of life help you find *'the Way'*.

In closing I would like to leave you with this timeless advice from chapter 8 of Lao Tsu's *Tao Te Ching*:

> *In life, be close to Nature.*
> *In thought, be profound.*
> *In relationships, be humane.*
> *In speech, be sincere.*

In ruling, be just.
In all things, be competent.
In action, seize the right time.

As William Ernest Henley wrote in *'Invictus'*:

'I am the master of my fate:
I am the captain of my soul'

There is hope. We have witnessed in our own lifetime the demise of communism in Russia, the demolition of the Berlin wall and the dismantling of Apartheid in South Africa.

Freedom, justice, respect and love will always overcome adversity. The great power of the human Spirit is undeniable and it only took one person to start the change. Surely, if we can overcome these momentous problems of the past we are capable of taking responsibility and control of our own health.

You can do it.

Thank you for reading this book.

The Golden Lion Academy

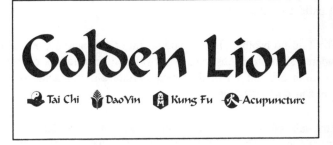

The Golden Lion Academy commenced operations in Melbourne, Australia in 1971. Since that time their membership has increased each year. One of the largest schools of Martial Arts in Australia, The Golden Lion Academy is regarded as one of the leaders in this discipline within the community.

Pier, Charles and Richard Tsui-Po, a family of three brothers, operate and run the Academy. With their traditional Chinese family background, they learnt their skills of both Chinese martial arts and healing from their ancestors. Since arriving in Australia, they have continued to increase and update their knowledge by studying regularly with many famous international experts. Together as The Golden Lion Academy, the three brothers form a formidable force in the martial arts industry. Their nephew, Steeve Kiat, now also at Master's level, teaches at the Academy with the family.

The Academy offers many associated services such as Kung Fu, Tai Chi, Self Defence as well as traditional Chinese medical science such as Acupuncture, Herbal medicine, Tui Na massage and Dao Yin.

Each of the three brothers specialises in a particular field of expertise. Charles is the principal Master of Tai Chi and Richard the principal Master of Kung Fu. Much of Pier's work today is in healing with traditional Chinese medicine. His articles on both health and martial arts are in constant demand by numerous magazines in Australia.

Pier is the founder of The Golden Lion Academy. He originally pioneered and taught Kung Fu in Melbourne. He learnt the ancient Dao Yin as a child and today he implements the modern Dao Yin into his clinic work with excellent patient results.

The Tsui-Po brothers head a large team of instructors that teach dedicated students all around Australia. They offer an instructor's course which includes both theory and practical training with the aim of teaching technique, philosophy and medicine together.

Hospitals, businesses and government departments are already successfully participating in The Golden Lion Academy classes and there is widespread interest in implementing these programmes further.

As the teachings of The Golden Lion Academy become better known within the community more and more people are taking advantage of the benefits derived from learning to heal themselves.

The Tsui-Po family continue their commitment to the development of human potential. They continue to teach people to develop greater inner strengths that build self-confidence, mental control and self-discipline whilst achieving peak mental and physical condition.

Pier Tsui-Po is available for seminars and workshops.

A video tape of the Dao Yin exercises is also available. Please contact The Golden Lion Academy's head office at:

2 Laser Drive, Rowville, Victoria, Australia, 3178

Bibliography

A treasury of the world's best loved poems, New York, Avenel Books, Crown Publishers, Inc., 1961.

Capra, Fritjof, *The Tao of Physics, An exploration of the parallels between modern physics and Eastern Mysticism*, Third edition, London, Flamingo, Harper Collins, 1992

Chan, Wing-Tsit, *A source book in Chinese Philosophy*, Fourth edition, Princetown, New Jersey, Princetown University Press, 1973

Palmer, Martin, *The Elements of Taoism*, Dorset, Great Britain, Element Books limited, 1991

Personal communications with various emminent practitioners of traditional chinese medicine and classical martial arts.

The Oxford Dictionary of Quotations, Third edition, Oxford, Oxford University Press, 1979

Thoreau, Henry David, *Walden*, New York, Avenel Books, Crown Publishers, Inc., 1973.

Veith, Ilza, *The Yellow Emperor's Classic of Internal Medicine*, New Edition, California, University of California Press Ltd, 1972